Download Your Ebook Today!

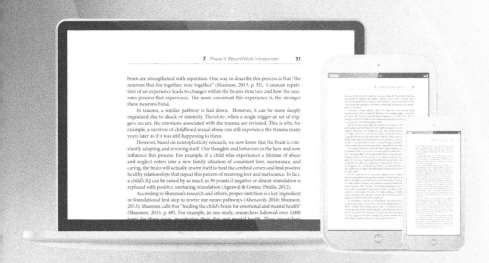

Your print purchase of *A Guide to Disseminating Your DNP Project* **includes an ebook download** to the device of your choice—increasing accessibility, portability, and searchability!

Download your ebook today at
http://spubonline.com/dnpproject
and enter the activation code below:

LSJE0CCDGF

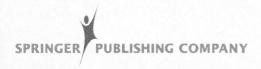

SPRINGER PUBLISHING COMPANY

springerpub.com

Marilyn Smith-Stoner, PhD, RN-BS, CNE, has been a nurse for more than 30 years. She began her career as a nurse in an associate degree program in Southern California. Her road to a doctorate took 20 years. She worked full time in many leadership positions during the entire time she was receiving her education. She benefited from many nontraditional programs aimed at ensuring that nurses who wanted to advance their education were able to so. Some of those programs included the consortium in the state of California university system, and an online doctoral program at the California Institute of Integral Studies in San Francisco, California. When the Internet was new, Dr. Stoner participated in one of the original online doctoral programs. In an era of dial-up modems and dot-matrix printers, she became an expert in educational technology while developing a program of scholarship and end-of-life care.

Dr. Smith-Stoner has more than 30 publications on end-of-life care, international travel, and many forms of technology. She has been a mentor to graduate students for more than 10 years. In her role as a volunteer nurse scientist, she has also assisted numerous students and clinicians in being published for the first time. This text is another in a series of guides that Dr. Smith-Stoner has created to advance nursing education and improve the care of patients everywhere.

A Guide to Disseminating Your DNP Project

Marilyn Smith-Stoner, PhD, RN-BS, CNE

SPRINGER PUBLISHING COMPANY

Springer Publishing Company, LLC
11 West 42nd Street
New York, NY 10036
www.springerpub.com

Acquisitions Editor: Joseph Morita
Senior Production Editor: Kris Parrish
Composition: S4Carlisle Publishing Services

ISBN: 978-0-8261-3316-8
ebook ISBN: 978-0-8261-3317-5
Faculty Guide ISBN: 978-0-8261-3461-5

Instructor's Materials: Qualified instructors may request supplements by emailing textbook@springerpub.com.

17 18 19 20/5 4 3 2 1

The author and the publisher of this Work have made every effort to use sources believed to be reliable to provide information that is accurate and compatible with the standards generally accepted at the time of publication. Because medical science is continually advancing, our knowledge base continues to expand. Therefore, as new information becomes available, changes in procedures become necessary. We recommend that the reader always consult current research and specific institutional policies before performing any clinical procedure. The author and publisher shall not be liable for any special, consequential, or exemplary damages resulting, in whole or in part, from the readers' use of, or reliance on, the information contained in this book. The publisher has no responsibility for the persistence or accuracy of URLs for external or third-party Internet websites referred to in this publication and does not guarantee that any content on such websites is, or will remain, accurate or appropriate.

Library of Congress Cataloging-in-Publication Data

Names: Smith-Stoner, Marilyn, author.
Title: A guide to disseminating your DNP project / Marilyn Smith-Stoner.
Other titles: Guide to disseminating your doctor of nursing practice project
Description: New York: Springer Publishing Company, [2018] | Includes
   bibliographical references.
Identifiers: LCCN 2017037022| ISBN 9780826133168 | ISBN 9780826134615
   (faculty guide) | ISBN 9780826133175 (ebook)
Subjects: | MESH: Information Dissemination--methods | Education, Nursing,
   Graduate | Nursing Research
Classification: LCC RT71 | NLM WY 18.5 | DDC 610.73071/1--dc23 LC record available at
https://lccn.loc.gov/2017037022

Contact us to receive discount rates on bulk purchases.
We can also customize our books to meet your needs.
For more information please contact: sales@springerpub.com

Printed in the United States of America.

This book is dedicated to all of the DNP students who are overwhelmed by the demands of life, their job, and advancing their education. All of us remember the difficulties of obtaining a doctorate. It is simply difficult. I've used the role modeling of my most beloved teacher to guide the creation of this text. Each and every doctoral student—indeed every nurse—has a story that others want to hear. No matter how difficult it may seem at the beginning of your journey, disseminating your capstone project is a very important final step for you. The final dissemination may be as simple as a letter to an editor advocating for health services in your community. It may be as profound as a screenplay highlighting the unique needs of the vulnerable populations of your area. You will find a method of sharing or disseminating your project that fits your interests. The world is waiting to hear what you did.

Contents

Unit IV: Disseminating Work via Oral Presentation Methods

Unit V: Disseminating Work via Art and Performance Methods

Unit VI: This Is the Beginning

Preface

This book is the most comprehensive resource for describing a multitude of methods of disseminating a doctor of nursing practice (DNP) capstone or other graduate-level project. No other publication includes explanations of how to use social media, web-based platforms, and artistic expressions such as poetry and music. Using the years of experience in producing webpages, blogs, multimedia, and other presentation material, you will find there is a wealth of information for most—beginner and experienced—users of 21st-century technology.

The text is divided into six units that begin with introducing new and traditional ways of disseminating DNP projects and proceeds to provide more in-depth explanations for each of the methods presented.

The reader will be taken on a journey that includes how to conduct press conferences, run publicity campaigns, find sources of television and radio outlets to be interviewed on, and use many other types of presentations. Throughout the process, readers are encouraged to consider not only developing an expertise in their subject matter but stepping outside their comfort zone to try a new educational method of teaching others about the results of their project and incorporating their passion for the subject matter.

Unit I begins with a general overview of the dissemination process and introduces a variety of possibilities to the reader.

Unit II continues to describe how to plan for dissemination methods well in advance of having to implement them.

Unit III focuses on dissemination strategies using print media. Unit IV focuses on oral presentation methods. Unit V explores nontraditional methods of dissemination utilizing a variety of arts including poetry, music, screenplays, and other forms of artistic expression. Unit VI concludes the textbook by focusing readers on incorporating the subject of the project and innovative method of delivery to enhance their career.

Throughout the process, the readers are provided with many specific resources to complete any of the methods presented. Nearly all of the recommended applications are free or have a free version. The depth and breadth of applications are sure to provide the reader with an exciting set of resources to choose from. **Qualified instructors may obtain access to an ancillary faculty guide by emailing textbook@springerpub.com.**

I am confident that the reader will be entertained, inspired, and satisfied with any dissemination project that is derived from the use of the tools and resources presented in this text.

Marilyn Smith-Stoner

CHAPTER 1

Why Take the Time to Disseminate Your Work?

☐ Chapter Checklist

☑	Your DNP project is a reflection of you and your hard work—there are many people who will benefit from your unique knowledge.
☑	Dissemination of your project is part of the nursing professional practice standard to continuously enhance and add to nursing art and science.
☑	Your project is the "voice" of the individuals who gave time, effort, and supported the work; disseminating respects and appreciates their contribution.
☑	Sharing your practice project enables you to join a community of practitioners who are part of a specific community of practitioners.
☑	Magnet® hospitals require specific contributions to clinical practice for advancement. Dissemination can contribute directly to your future occupational success.
☑	Dissemination is a requirement of the nursing accreditation agencies for your program.

With the ubiquitous presence of technology, dissemination of all types of information is now part of our daily lives. We have the ability to share the most trivial information at our fingertips. We also have the power to shape the way our friends, families, and communities perceive an important health issue or react to a disaster. With each "share" of information we sow seeds, which is what the word *dissemination* means. As you progress through your DNP program, you will identify a topic, explore its significance, and shape its presentation using systematic scientific methods within a learning community.

Growing the knowledge base of nursing is a shared responsibility of all nurses, especially doctorally prepared nurses, who are testing knowledge generated by others and shaping nursing practice by systematically applying research to many practice settings. When the research needs to be adapted to a unique situation or population, a DNP graduate knows how to go about making adjustments and providing feedback to the original researchers to help them further develop their ideas. In this ongoing, ever-expanding feedback loop, the process of sharing, sowing new seeds of knowledge, brings us closer to our goal of preventing avoidable illness and injury, enhancing quality of life, and comforting those who have come to the end of life.

Throughout the process, you are gathering insights to be shared. Some you will keep; others will be discarded. Tracking the process of developing your ideas is the heart of scholarly process. The process is dynamic and creative. Within the community of learners on the journey with you are your DNP student colleagues, faculty, educational leaders, clinician colleagues and clients, patients, and community members of all types. They all have a vested interest in knowing what the results of your shared work are. Every part of your DNP project means something to the people involved; they have part of the ownership through their participation.

The sharing of personal information to people, known and unknown, who share specific interests is the same as disseminating information to other professions that serve the same individuals who were incorporated into your project. Without sharing, without growing nursing art and science, health care workers, patients, and those who love them lose out on benefiting on what you've done. No one has considered the problem, solution, and combination of context and analysis like you have. Letting others know what you did, what worked, and what did not is a matter of life or death to some group of people.

By sharing your data, experience, insights, lessons learned, and suggestions for the future, you move the problem and nursing along. The project is not completed until the discussion of it is widely shared with others in the field.

Completing a DNP project is something only a few nurses accomplish in a lifetime. In 2015, there were just over 26,000 graduates and students in DNP programs, or about 8% of nurses! All DNP graduates need to disseminate the products of their projects to make a significant impact on nursing care.

☐ Contributions to Nursing Art and Science

The doctorate of nursing practice projects present a unique opportunity to advance nursing art and science, only if the information is presented beyond the university where the degree was obtained. Nursing science has been built through a continuous process of adding to what is known, helping to eliminate the knowledge that is no longer supported in evidence, and pointing the way to future areas where nursing needs to focus. There are many gaps that remain in nursing knowledge and much work left to do.

☐ Your Project Is the "Voice" of Others

Many individuals participated in your project. Disseminating your project gives voice to the individuals who contributed their insights, energy, and other resources to ensure your success. As a result, dissemination of your unique application of knowledge gained from their energy is the other side of the partnership you established with them. Sharing your work means their identities, needs, and self-awareness may be known by the rest of society.

☐ Establishes Your Expertise

The project you complete will be infused with your ideas, knowledge, values, and experiences. You will be changed by the process and have the opportunity to change the way others view your topic. The population you select, the clinical issue you identify, the collection of prior research, and the application of evidence will be unique to you. You may find that you have developed a new model of care, pointed out the gaps in existing knowledge, or found a solution to a problem that was not known prior to your work. No one will be able to benefit from your efforts without being able to access your work. Someone else may get credit; someone who took the time to disseminate their work using your ideas will get the credit if they are the first to tell others about what they learned.

☐ Contribute to Your Career Goals

Many DNPs will find that their employer rewards an advanced degree directly with a raise or changed role. Some will attain leadership positions with increased wages as a result of a new degree earned (Terhaar, Taylor, & Sylvia, 2016). Magnet hospitals generally reward staff who contribute to scholarship financially and organizationally. Each agency will have its own unique requirements. Make sure you speak with leaders in your organization to know how you can tap into higher positions/income at your agency as a result of your work. The emphasis on dissemination is a common requirement of advancement at Magnet hospitals.

☐ Required by Accrediting Agencies

Sustainability is an important component of any program. By readily fulfilling the accreditation requirements that your DNP program must meet, you are contributing to the sustainability of the program. DNP programs are on the rise. Accreditation is an important part of ensuring the program remains healthy for future students.

☐ Specifics of Disseminating Your DNP Project

There are many models to follow to disseminate your project. One such contemporary model is the SHARED model, explained in the text that follows.

Select the topic or seeds of nursing knowledge you want to plant and nurture. Your ideas will change from the beginning to the end of the program. That's the nature of evidence-based practice. As new knowledge is generated, practice that is no longer supported by evidence is phased out. Helping to phase out ineffective practice is an important part of disseminating your work. By helping colleagues, the public, and leaders in the field understand what doesn't work anymore and why, you clear a path for new and better methods. Provide both clear evidence for new practice and deconstruct the effectiveness of existing practice.

Habits need to be developed that are effective and time efficient. Many students are already caregivers of their own families, parents, full-time workers in addition to full-time students. Without a significant change in daily habits it is difficult to work effectively and complete work on time. Students are remarkable in what they are able to do! By following the SHARED model, it is possible to take on the considerable work of a DNP degree and stay focused along the way.

Assessing the current knowledge base in your field is the place to begin the DNP process. Next assess the study skills, technology skills, and the knowledge and skills you must develop, in addition to determining your budget and the program that suits you. Just like patient care, assessment is the first place to start to ensure that effort is focused on the correct actions.

Recording of work, thoughts, and progress done continuously throughout your program is critical to your success. It is also necessary to be able to demonstrate ownership of your ideas. Keeping records of what you are doing, what you need to do, and how you will accomplish all of what you have to do is part of forming doctoral habits, which also lower your stress level and keep you on track.

Enthusiasm throughout the process—you are the best champion of your own work. Keeping your enthusiasm up means you keep your project a priority. As a caregiver and leader, many people are asking for you time. Keep those around you informed of your work and let them know how important it is to you and to others.

Dissemination involves spreading information into public spaces for the people who can most benefit from knowing the information. For decades, this meant publishing articles in professional journals with rigid author guidelines. Not anymore. Dissemination can take many forms: the traditional print publication is no longer emphasized in the American Association of Colleges of Nursing (AACN) Essentials for the DNP (2006). Newer, digital forms of dissemination are suggested (Table 1.1). Other forms, often tailored to the audience who most

TABLE 1.1 Types of Dissemination of DNP Work

Print	Presentation
Peer-reviewed journal Review of the literature for an article, project, or practice, or policy change	Scholarly presentation at professional meetings
Publications in professional publications such as newsletters and special reports	Continuing-education presentations for professionals Innovative instructional methods for students
Organizational policies and procedures Website content Budgetary analysis; review of systems processes and outcomes	Continuing education for staff, benefactors, and volunteers Bulletin boards in public locations
Health education material for the public	Presentations at support groups for specific conditions, wellness presentations for community groups
Letters to the editor, letters to elected representatives on health issues	Testimony at public meetings
Digital media	
Blogs, websites maintained	Videos—YouTube, Vimeo Maintain a board on Pinterest Page on Facebook Twitter feed
Social media: Facebook, Twitter, Instagram, Tumblr, Reddit	SlideShare Infographics
eBooks and other electronic media	Public domain photos in repositories
Broadcast	
Social media streaming Periscope Blab Facebook streaming Google Hangouts	Television interviews Radio interviews Podcast interviews Podcasts
Performances	
Poetry Fiction Drawing Photography exhibit	Theater performances Songs

(continued)

TABLE 1.1 **Types of Dissemination of DNP Work** (*continued*)

Print	Presentation
Other	
Grant applications Quality reports	Travel project to apply principles in the field
Reflective and process oriented	
Description of process of preparing, completing DNP Return on investment Return on expectations	Lessons learned regarding: Working, getting an education, having a family What happened after the degree? Was it worth it?

needs and wants to hear what you have to say, such as blogs, videos, social media chats/streams, games, press conferences, consultation services, public advocacy, specialized lesson plans, and educational programs are just a few of the limitless possibilities. Program resources, and especially faculty availability, are important considerations (Dols, Hernández, & Miles, 2016).

If you are considering publishing some or all of your work in a nursing journal, focus on a clinical journal that appeals to nurses working at the bedside in the specialty area that relates to your topic. Table 1.2 lists a selection of work by BSN and MSN students that was published. By breaking up sections of your capstone work, you can find subtopics within your overall project that may make excellent articles. Speak with your advisor about how to transform an academic assignment into a publishable paper. Never send an assignment turned in for a grade to a professional journal expecting it to be reviewed for publication. The paper will only be reviewed if it complies with the author guidelines of the journal. These guidelines are available on the journal website. How to submit an article for publication will be covered later in the book in much more detail. As you read journal articles for assignments in your classes, take note of journals that resonate with you. If you decide to submit an article for publication, you may find the journals you regularly read are the best ones to consider for your own articles.

Your capstone journal will be a complete record of your journey to complete the DNP degree. Your understanding of advanced nursing practice and your research topic will transform from a vague notion to a detailed description of a problem and ultimately a solution to the problem you identified. Your topic may focus on a specific population, a unique health care condition(s), a new bundle of patient care interventions, or the difference between day- and night-shift care outcomes, for example. The possibilities for how you will develop the project are endless.

TABLE 1.2 Select List of Dr. Stoner's Students' Publications

1	Baca, K., Rico, M., & Stoner, M. (2015). Embracing technology to strengthen care and enhance human connection. *Dimensions of Critical Care Nursing, 34*(3), 179–180. doi:10.1097/DCC.0000000000000111
2	Marcial, L., Brazina, M., Diaz, A., Jaramillo, C., Marentes, G., & Mazmanian, N. (2013). A brief article. Is this the cost of caring? A student perspective on compassion fatigue. *Dimensions of Critical Care Nursing, 32*(1), 18–21. doi:10.1097/DCC.0b013e31826bc687
3	Gardiner, K., Mistretta, D., Rader, B., & Walker, K. (2013). Student research. A brief report: A mere toothbrush or a brilliant lifesaver? *Dimensions of Critical Care Nursing, 32*(1), 33–35. doi:10.1097/DCC.0b013e31827682ce
4	Rose, C., Bonn, A., MacDonald, K., & Avila, S. (2012). Interdisciplinary education on discussing end-of-life care. *Dimensions of Critical Care Nursing, 31*(4), 236–240. doi:10.1097/DCC.0b013e318256d808
5	Bajer, L. (2012). Personal reflection. *Dimensions of Critical Care Nursing, 31*(5), 287–289.
6	Van, H., Chang, S., Olivas, R., Almacen, C., Dimanlig, M., & Rodriguez, H. (2012). A student paper. *Dimensions of Critical Care Nursing, 31*(6), 318–321. doi:10.1097/DCC.0b013e31826bc7f7

In the DNP Essentials (2006), the AACN describes the DNP program as preparing graduates to collaborate, communicate, lead, and systematically work to make positive changes in society. DNP education is meant to help graduates achieve the highest level of clinical practice. Throughout your program you have been an artist who shapes knowledge in unique ways through your verbal, written, reflective, and other assignments. Only you can tell the story of the people who were the focus of your practice-based project.

As you develop your knowledge of how to apply research to create evidence-based care models, you become what the AACN (2015) envisions for the role of the DNP. Events and knowledge of health care trends continuously shape the understanding of the DNP role. Rapid growth in the capacity to educate DNP nurses has led to a need to evaluate the evolution of the culminating project required by all programs. AACN encourages DNP programs to urge graduates to incorporate all types of traditional, digital, innovative, and creative ways of spreading the knowledge gained from their projects. In these early years of the DNP, the focus has been on applying traditional methods of dissemination to this new degree, which hasn't worked as well as it could.

This book is a direct result of listening to editors of nursing journals describe the difficulty of receiving hundreds of academically prepared project papers that were ill suited to be considered for peer review, let alone publication. In years to come, it is fitting that DNP programs not only require dissemination well beyond a print publication. Instead, the true success of a DNP program will be transformed from using submissions for publication as a mark of success, to measuring acceptance rates for publication, downloads of podcasts, shares in social media, testimony to policy makers, arts of all kinds, and likely, many methods yet to be developed. The DNP graduate of the 21st century will be able to utilize many forms of technology to spread the knowledge gained from each and every practice project. Table 1.1 listed some examples of what you can start thinking about. Table 1.3 gives specific examples of nurses who are using these technologies in some way. The idea is to become a consumer of these technologies. By subscribing to podcasts, in other words, developing another new habit, you will be able to

TABLE 1.3 Examples of Innovative Presentations of Health Content

	Traditional	Virtual
Manuscript/Publication	X	
Blogs: Nurse Keith, www.nursekeith.com		X
Podcasts: Elizabeth Scala, https://elizabethscala.com/podcast-2		X
Twitter: We Communities, http://wecommunities.org/resources/twitterversity		X
Websites: NerdyNurse, https://thenerdynurse.com		X
Artwork: Art By Nurses	X	
Fiction: *No Other Medicine*, www.gailhallas.com	X	X
eBook: *Echo Heron*, www.echoheron.com		X
Letter to the Editor: Theresa Brown	X	
Testimony at public hearing: Workplace violence	X	
Infographic: Nightingale		X
Community organizing: COPAR Model	X	
Professional practice committee work	X	
Fund-raiser: 2013 Rose Parade Float	X	X

TABLE 1.3 **Examples of Innovative Presentations of Health Content** (*continued*)

	Traditional	Virtual
Innovative academic course work: Nurse Tim	✕	✕
Active learning through simulation: National League for Nursing	✕	

Expert professional consultation:
  Grant writing: Kate Angilly
  Expert consultant: Brenda Pratt Shafer
  Test-item writing: NCLEX
	✕	

Art:
  Poetry: *A Fence or an Ambulance* (Exhibit 1.1)
  Scrubs collection of poetry
    Theater: Anna Deavere Smith
    Music: Deb Gauldin
  Literature
    Theater: Bonnie Hunt
    Table reading scripts: Suzanne Gordon
    Puppet other shows: Teaching Diabetes Care
    Craft: Paula White
    Painting: *American Journal of Nursing* Description
	✕	✕

better assess whether this medium is right for your own use. The same is true for reading blogs, creating videos, and the other technologies listed. Each will be covered in the book and it's up to you to select not only your capstone topic, but the method(s) that you will use to tell the world about what you have done.

This book bridges traditional views of disseminating new knowledge via print and suggests knowledge may be spread using many forms of digital media, all types of arts, advocacy, and education. As you proceed through the program, take note of the types of information you enjoy and gravitate to. Ask the people with whom you come in contact how they get information and find entertainment. You will find the best way to develop your own dissemination strategy by incorporating what is relevant to the people who are the focus of your project using the informational sources they use.

Start Thinking About Dissemination on Day 1

Although dissemination is the last thing you do in your program, think about how you might achieve it when you start your program. Each program sets its own standard for disseminating the work of graduate students that needs to be followed. It can take time to improve your existing skills or to learn new skills so start experimenting with new technology as you complete individual assignments.

By the end of your DNP education, you will be exposed to many new methods you can use to disseminate your work. Practice using these methods, most of which can be done from a mobile device, in small ways. Try making a sound recording, making a video, creating a personal logo that brands your work to you as an individual. This book will present many examples of how to disseminate scholarship so that it will reach your intended audience in the best possible way—to have the greatest impact.

☐ DNP Projects

In their white paper of August 2015, "The Doctor of Nursing Practice: Current Issues and Clarifying Recommendations," the AACN issued a clarification on the current state of the DNP degree. The clarification of the scholarly focus of the DNP was among the many items described. According to AACN:

> DNP programs focus on the translation of new science, its application and evaluation. The report goes on to say graduates are prepared to generate new knowledge through innovation of practice change, the translation of evidence, and the implementation of quality improvement processes in specific practice settings, systems, or with specific populations to improve health or health outcomes. (2015, p. 2)

This clarification of the focus of the DNP also opens up many possibilities for dissemination. Although publication in a peer-reviewed journal is almost the singular standard for a research-based doctorate, a DNP is open to any activity that is scholarly and is relevant to the population that is the focus of the project. For example, a project that focuses on raising teenagers' awareness of sexual health may best be conducted using a stage play, multimedia event, or creating a short explanatory videos rather than creating a brochure with printed words.

Using innovation to present important health care information is not a new idea. Many innovative DNP projects are described in the text by Anderson, Knestrick, and Barroso (2014).

Read the brilliant poem "A Fence or an Ambulance", presented in Exhibit 1.1. It is entertaining, poignant, humorous, and very relevant to nursing and current trends in prevention, even though it was written by Joseph Malin in 1895. Becoming familiar with this classic poet may help you begin to "think outside the box" as you consider both the focus of your project and the closely related topic of how you will provide the information you assemble to the audience outside your program.

As you proceed through the program, think creatively about dissemination and speak with your faculty advisor about it. Ensure your dissemination plan is consistent with the program guidelines. If you encounter any reluctance to adaptation of dissemination methods, refer your student representative or the faculty to the 2015 AACN white paper mentioned earlier.

☐ The Impact of Digital Communication

Understanding the opportunities and barriers to communicating digitally while developing your project helps focus and prepare you to shape the message and

EXHIBIT 1.1 **A Fence or an Ambulance**

Twas a dangerous cliff, as they freely confessed,
though to walk near its crest was so pleasant;
but over its terrible edge there had slipped
a duke and full many a peasant.
So the people said something would have to be done,
but their projects did not at all tally;
some said, 'Put a fence 'round the edge of the cliff,'
some, 'An ambulance down in the valley.'
But the cry for the ambulance carried the day,
for it spread through the neighboring city;
a fence may be useful or not, it is true,
but each heart became full of pity
for those who slipped over the dangerous cliff;
And the dwellers in highway and alley
gave pounds and gave pence, not to put up a fence,
but for an ambulance down in the valley.
'For the cliff is all right, if you're careful,' they said,
'and if folks even slip and are dropping,
it isn't the slipping that hurts them so much
as the shock down below when they're stopping.'
So day after day, as these mishaps occurred,
quick forth would those rescuers sally
to pick up the victims who fell off the cliff,
with their ambulance down in the valley.
Then an old sage remarked: 'It's a marvel to me
that people give far more attention
to repairing results than to stopping the cause,
when they'd much better aim at prevention.
Let us stop at its source all this mischief,' cried he,
'come, neighbors and friends, let us rally;
if the cliff we will fence, we might almost dispense
with the ambulance down in the valley.'

— *Joseph Malins*

the method of disseminating your new knowledge. Whatever you produce will probably be consumed via a mobile digital device such as your phone. The content may come in the form of text, audio, video, images, or a combination of all four components. Forms of "digital knowing" open up the universe of knowledge to anyone with access to the Internet, cable, or other media, some of which is presented in a small number of characters (such as Twitter), or on a small screen, such as the 2 to 6 inches available on a phone. It is essential to understand the limitations presented by social media providers *and* the device where the end product of your dissemination will be consumed as they profoundly influence each other.

The relationship of content and method of presentation is difficult to separate because the access to digital content is actually rewiring our brains. Sohlberg and Mateer's (1987) model of attention describes the three levels of attention we have developed: sustained, selective, and alternating. In their research on 2,000 Canadians performing different activities while being studied using standard neurofunctional methods, the researchers found that participants' ability to remain focused on a task was in part related to social media usage. In short, the more social media the user consumed, the shorter the attention span of the user. Compared with television viewers, who can process information more effectively, social media users tend to lose interest quickly. As you begin your program of study, take note of your own attention span. Maintain a journal detailing your insight into how you learn best. Make a note of how people in your project learn and what types of technology they use.

Technology is changing rapidly and you cannot master all the new possibilities to creatively present your work. Traditionally, doctoral students choose their committee based on their content expertise. This is less common in DNP programs, where students are already experts in their field. Consider finding a committee that has dissemination expertise. If your project is focused on improving access to care, then seek out someone for your committee with that experience. Identify committee members who have testified on behalf of others, are sought out for interviews by news organizations, or have other expertise. Use social media to understand how your program faculty can provide you with the dissemination help you will need. If you are planning on submitting an article for publication, use a committee that can help you shape a relevant, timely, and innovative article for a publication that is a best fit for you and the people who need to know what you've done. DNP dissemination methods should reflect the scholarship of your degree, not just a checkmark on an application for graduation.

The essence of the project is knowledge gained; the method you choose to disseminate the project will have a huge impact on the accessibility of your new knowledge to the people who could most benefit from knowing about your work. The purpose of describing some specific methods of dissemination in this chapter is to encourage and inspire you to think about the future to ensure your efforts will remain relevant, useful, and available to others interested in the same subject you choose.

A short list of possible new dissemination methods is presented in Table 1.1. In the past, print methods, such as article, books, brochure, and other print media, have been emphasized. This is no longer the case, as emphasized by the AACN's white paper of 2015. In 2017 and beyond, a research-based article in a nursing journal can now be transformed into a graphic novel, formerly known as a *comic book*. If teenagers or young adults are the focus of your project, they may benefit more from a superhero describing how to let an adult know they need help with a personal issue, than a booklet full of words that may or may not be understood.

Before selecting new methods of dissemination, check with your advisor and follow the university's guidelines. As mentioned, you may need to learn a new skill(s), such as creating videos, which will require a storyboard, similar to an outline done for a paper, in order to create a quality project. Print displays, such as scholarly posters, will require synthesizing; you must significantly condense your project paper from thousands of words to a few hundred. Editing your own work can be difficult so you may need help. Reach out to experts in graphic design, editing, and other skills as necessary.

Text-Based Presentation Types

For decades, the standard of presenting information has been publication in books and journals as well as newsletters and official reports. Concise summaries of content have been presented in real time to classes of students and others through PowerPoint presentations given at conferences. These methods of presenting information have an important place in the transmission of information. Conferences, especially those clinicians go to for updates on the newest evidence, have the potential to significantly affect patient care. Clinicians are more likely to read information in clinically focused journals than research-focused ones (Oermann, Shaw-Kokot, Knafl, & Dowell, 2010). It follows that conferences practitioners come to for professional development will have a direct benefit in patient care.

Traditional methods of dissemination focus on both peer-reviewed publications and presentations at nursing and other conferences. Both options offer many variations. The many printed forms of dissemination in peer-reviewed articles in scholarly journals take about a year to produce, from submission, to published product. Newer methods provide interesting and aesthetically engaging ways of presenting prioritized information, however. A primary method used today is aninfographic.

Table 1.2 lists student publications from an undergraduate research course. The list is provided to demonstrate that there are many types of articles that those used to present primary research generally thought of as doctoral work. You may consider submitting an article on "lessons learned," tips for getting a DNP, or stories of challenge and triumph in the very busy life of doctoral students, who often have families, provide care to aging elders, and work at demanding jobs. Personal-experience articles are highly sought after and popular. Remember that reading and complying with author guidelines is the most effective way to get the journal to consider your topic. Understanding the importance of following author guidelines cannot be overstated.

Other forms of printed dissemination include a new brochure with educational content, a newsletter article written for a professional association, and many more. Operational documents, such as a budget analysis, a special report detailing a new service, or other methods of evaluation of a clinical care process can also be used.

Transforming clinical care processes for customers served by your agency are particularly noteworthy. Helping patients and their families understand hospital procedures, such as the functions of the interdisciplinary team, what to expect after discharge to home, how to recognize signs of both improvement and decline, are significant contributions to nursing knowledge.

Another category of dissemination methods focuses on informing and educating the public. Letters to the editor, press releases, and articles intended for the public can reach beyond people not directly affected by the topic of your project. Your published work designed for members of the general public can be the start of a movement to address hunger, disease, or other social issues facing the patients of your facility.

☐ Traditional Oral Presentations

Oral presentations at educational conferences are commonly made by graduate students. Other presentations can be done at community conferences, for elected officials, or other interested groups. At the minimum, you should plan to present your findings to the people involved in helping you with the project. The oral presentation can be done from a podium or in conjunction with a poster (Christenbery & Latham, 2013).

☐ Digital Content

Websites, blogs, and other social media effectively present your material to a large number of people. They are inexpensive and fairly straightforward to create. Start with the social media you use and find influencers in the areas of your interest. Each time you find an expert in your subject, research his or her publications *and* social media accounts, podcasts, and other digital media such as interviews Table 1.1 provides a list of many different types of ways to disseminate portions and your final comprehensive capstone work. All of these resources have the potential to provide you with content from the specialists you may be using in your project.

☐ Traditional Web and Hybrid Dissemination

The Iowa Model is a traditional model of dissemination that has been used successfully in DNP programs (Lloyd, D'Errico, & Bristol, 2016). To explore the possibilities of dissemination, consume multiple types of media in your area of interest. Consuming select types of media in a variety of formats will help you to understand where experts are and how they present their specialties. For example, consider Suzanne Gordon (www.suzannecgordon.com), world-renowned journalist who is both a critic of and advocate for nursing. Her books are impressive; her classic (co-written), *From Silence to Voice: What Nurses Know and Must Communicate to the Public (The Culture and Politics of Health Care Work)* (Buresh & Godron, 2013) will help you develop expertise in areas where specific audiences consume content. Through Ms. Gordon's presence in social media—Twitter and Facebook—you can speak directly to her. Through her website you can easily find her social media accounts and keep up with her work. Her example is one that can be a springboard for brainstorming what you can do. Deciding what you will eventually do will be based on your program requirements, assessment activities, and data you collect and you can use information from nursing science to guide the process (Riner, 2015).

You'll learn how to craft content to meet the interests of consumers, who can be anyone from professionals to members of the public with a personal interest in a subject. While you are mastering the prescribed content of your program steadily, build up the social media that you consume.

Much of social media is formatted as microblogs, where content is short, concise, and distributed over platforms such as Twitter. Other social media postings can be longer, such as those appearing on Facebook, Google Plus, and Instagram. However, they are all much shorter than a published paper. Web content is always focused on addressing a specific issue rather than an in-depth comprehensive description of a topic done for academic audiences.

Hybrid approaches to disseminating information may combine a series of shorter videos, postings, or other material. The program requirements will help you determine what type and quantity of material qualifies for meeting graduation requirements. When you first start to develop your knowledge and skill in new methods of knowledge creation and dissemination, read and curate to collect information first. You can use expert social media content in your own work, too. Follow the formatting guidelines required by your university when including this media in your assignments.

☐ First Steps

Whether you are new to social media or an experienced consumer or creator, use your program's graduation requirements, your knowledge of where leaders in the subject are presenting their ideas, and this book to develop a relevant plan for dissemination of your project. The first few chapters of this book are meant to open the door to considering dissemination alternatives that are most relevant to the people who need to hear about your project. Even if you have not decided on a topic for your project and have never used social media, start to consume three or four types of media in a topic you do care about. Two of the most common topics on the Internet are cats and recipes. If you have an interest in either, and have not yet determined your project area, start by finding influencers or experts in either of these two areas, so you can develop new digital skills.

Using the content you create in papers, online postings, posters, and presentations, you can develop core content that can be transformed into a series of tweets in Twitter; short videos uploaded to YouTube, Vimeo, or other platform; and other types of media. Table 1.3 provides a brief list of innovative digital media produced by nurses for nurses and the public. The transformed content will become part of a vast supply of material that can be used to create anything from a letter to the editor on an important health issue to an updated policy and procedure at your organization.

Data collection is an ongoing process of assessing, critiquing, and sorting the usable from the unusable. Data collection often begins in the college library. However, the search is never over and includes collecting digital content such as social media, podcasts, videos, and other methods of dissemination the authors of prior work you are interested in are producing. Set up accounts in forums where the experts are talking online. Nearly all are free and as easy to disconnect as they are to subscribe to.

The first step in the long process of obtaining your DNP starts with the time-tested activities of all DNP students, which are to read, discuss, and analyze how the basics of advanced practice nursing relate to your area of interest. Once you start analyzing research and evidence and receive formal and informal feed-back on your ideas, you can start producing your own content. I encourage you to share your early ideas publicly via social media and let others who are interested in your topic respond to your work.

Your faculty cannot be experts in the topic of every single student in their classes. This will be an important way for you to be mentored by content experts. One concept advanced practice nurses learn is that there is an endless combination of patient and family care challenges and as such there is a need to tap into as big a supply of knowledge as possible. There is no bigger supply of knowledge than the open Internet of information.

Group Projects

You may choose to do your project with another person. I completed my dissertation project with another doctoral student (Smith-Stoner & Weber, 2000). There are positives and negatives to completing something as important as your final project with one or more people. Check with your faculty advisor and program handbook about the possibility of a group project and the requirements for it. We enjoyed working together as we experienced the expected stresses and strains. You will want to think long and hard about who you pick and have a serious conversation about life goals with this person. Because health care is inherently a team activity, at least consider exploring a collaborative project.

☐ Conclusions

You will find an exciting collection of dissemination methods discussed throughout this text. I have used them and find they work well. Even if your program requires a submission of an article for publication, you will still get help in this text (Unit III). If you think you cannot get published—you are wrong. Table 1.2 shows you that with proper preparation it is possible to begin publishing as a student. Nursing journals also regularly publish poetry, photographic essays, short stories and art; whatever your interest and talents, there is a place in print or on the web for your work.

REFERENCES

American Association of Colleges of Nursing. (2006). *The essentials of doctoral education for advanced nursing practice*. Retrieved from http://www.aacnnursing.org/DNP/DNP-Essentials

American Association of Colleges of Nursing. (2015). *The doctor of nursing practice: Current issues and clarifying recommendations*. Retrieved from http://www.aacnnursing.org/Portals/42/DNP/DNP-Implementation.pdf?ver=2017-08-01-105830-517

Anderson, B. A., Knestrick, J. M., & Barroso, R. (2014). *DNP capstone projects: Exemplars of excellence in practice*. New York, NY: Springer Publishing.

Buresh, B., & Godron, S. (2013). *From silence to voice: What nurses know and must communicate to the public (The culture and politics of health care work)* (3rd ed.). Ithaca, NY: ILR Press.

Christenbery, T. L., & Latham, T. G. (2013). Creating effective scholarly posters: A guide for DNP students. *Journal of the American Association of Nurse Practitioners, 25*(1), 16–23. doi:10.1111/j.1745-7599.2012.00790.x

Dols, J. D., Hernández, C., & Miles, H. (2016). The DNP project: Quandaries for nursing scholars. *Nursing Outlook, 65*(1), 84–93. doi:10.1016/j.outlook.2016.07.009

Lloyd, S. T., D'Errico, E., & Bristol, S. T. (2016). Use of the Iowa Model of Research in Practice as a curriculum framework for doctor of nursing practice (DNP) project completion. *Nursing Education Perspectives, 37*(1), 51–53. doi:10.5480/14-1364

Oermann, M., Shaw-Kokot, J., Knafl, G., & Dowell, J. (2010). Dissemination of research into clinical nursing literature. *Journal of Clinical Nursing, 19*(23/24), 3435–3442. doi:10.1111/j.1365-2702.2010.03427.x

Riner, M. E. (2015). Using implementation science as the core of the doctor of nursing practice inquiry project. *Journal of Professional Nursing, 31*, 200–207.

Smith-Stoner, M., & Weber, T. (2000). *Developing theory using emergent inquiry: A study of meaningful online learning for women* (Doctoral dissertation). San Francisco: California Institute of Integral Studies.

Sohlberg, M. M., & Mateer, C. A. (1987). Effectiveness of an attention-training program. *Journal of Clinical and Experimental Neuropsychology, 9*(2), 117–130.

Terhaar, M. F., Taylor, L. A., & Sylvia, M. L. (2016). The doctor of nursing practice: From start-up to impact. *Nursing Education Perspectives, 37*(1), 3–9. doi:10.5480/14-1519

CHAPTER 2

Clarifying Research-Focused or Practice-Focused Scholarship

☐ Chapter Checklist

☑	Describe practice scholarship.
☑	Describe research scholarship.
☑	Describe quality-improvement projects.
☑	Describe translational of research.

☐ Sharing Scholarship

As you are planning to introduce yourself to the profession of nursing as a practice-focused scholar, you will have a lot of decisions to make. Take a breath and reflect on the importance of open sharing and how, topic by topic, nursing has advanced as a profession. Florence Nightingale's *Notes on Nursing* were just records of observations she kept about what worked and didn't work. You will also be doing this. By sharing your observations, activities, and self-critique of what worked and what did not, you build the profession up. When nurses with a DNP and other degrees of scholarship build the knowledge base, everyone benefits from the work.

Benefit comes from sharing what worked and what *didn't* work. Consumers of the products of your doctoral work want what you want: an honest, usable, and relevant description of a meaningful project. With technology, you can choose to share your project one step at a time or all at once. Consider the needs of the people who will most benefit from reading your work. Some subjects, like policies and procedures, don't work well when shared a section at a time. Many procedures are too complicated or lengthy to share in pieces. Others, like the development of video, start with a concept, proceed to sketches and descriptions of what will be done, then a script is written, and finally a recording is made. Even after a recording, there is postproduction work. "Showing your work" as you proceed along the process gives the maximum number of people an opportunity to give you feedback. Continuous feedback makes your DNP project stronger and more likely to benefit a wider group of colleagues, patients, and others.

As you develop, your project follows the SHARED model. The **S** of SHARED, refers to selecting the topic, which is the first step. Most doctoral projects will be focused on a subject that is practice based and applies existing information, rather than answering a question about a topic when the answer is unknown or not well understood. The differences are described in the text that follows. The topic and the method of defining your topic are difficult to separate, so I include them together.

☐ Types of Scholarship

Research/discovery and practice-based scholarship are the two primary types of scholarship discussed in this text. Practice-based scholarship is the primary method of scholarship presented. However, one cannot exist without the other. They are derived and flow from each other naturally and are mutually interdependent. Nursing research scholarship begins with a desire to understand why something does not work well and needs to be addressed. It can also begin with an appreciation for what works really well and a desire to replicate a successful result. A gap in knowledge or need to expand the population of people included in research also tends to favor a traditional research study. A practice-based project will apply the information already gathered. This chapter will help you clarify the important differences. I encourage you to adopt the key terms and phrases used in this chapter to keep your communication to others clear about the type of project you are doing.

If you find the distinction between discovery/research and practice-based or translational research confusing, you are not alone. Many nursing programs, research review boards, researchers, and health care agencies have struggled with making a distinction between research studies and nonresearch or practice-based projects (see Table 2.1).

The DNP white paper from the American Association of Colleges of Nursing (AACN, 2015) describes the current focus of the culminating project in nursing education:

> Graduates of both research- and practice-focused doctoral programs are prepared to generate new knowledge. However, research-focused graduates are prepared to generate knowledge through rigorous research and statistical methodologies that may be broadly applicable or generalizable; practice-focused graduates are prepared to generate new knowledge through innovation of practice change, the translation of evidence, and the implementation of quality improvement processes in specific practice settings, systems, or with specific populations to improve health or health

outcomes. New knowledge generated through practice innovation, for example, could be of value to other practice settings. This new knowledge is considered transferrable but is not considered generalizable. (p. 2)

Many programs incorporate the work of Boyer (1990) to further define practice scholarship. Simply put, clinicians are in the best place to be the role model to apply research, using knowledge of evidence-based practice. Practice scholars and DNP graduates provide service to an organization through engaging others to improve care outcomes, institutional processes, or practices while providing ongoing education to others through their work on the ground in the clinical area.

TABLE 2.1 Examples of Research-Focused or Practice-Focused Scholarship

Research-Focused Scholarship	Practice-Focused Scholarship
Fike, G. C. (2015). Augmenting survey completion and rates of returns for patients with low literacy: A randomized control trial of telephone follow-up. *International Journal Nursing Clinical Practice, 2*, 154.	Krebbeks, V. P., & Cunningham, V. M. (2013). A DNP nurse-managed hepatitis C clinic, improving quality of life for those in a rural area. *Online Journal of Rural Nursing & Health Care, 13*(1), 127–148.
McGrath, C. (2014). The use of fresh whole blood and its effect on survival rates in massive trauma: Review of a war trauma database. Retrieved from https://nursing.vanderbilt.edu/images/dnp/scholarly/2014/colonel_caroline_mcgrath_researchposter.jpg	Hathaway, D., Jacob, S., Stegbauer, C., Thompson, C., & Graff, C. (2006). The practice doctorate: Perspectives of early adopters. *Journal of Nursing Education, 45*(12), 487–496.
	Jahner, J. (2015). Palliative care: Patient-centered assessment and communication to improve quality of life. *New Mexico Nurse, 60*(4), 4–6.
	Hart, J. L., & Braband, B. (2015). Doctor of Nursing Practice, practice improvement project: A simulation-based emergency preparedness program in immediate care. *Clinical Scholars Review, 8*(2), 201–207. doi:10.1891/1939-2095.8.2.201
	Hodges, H. C. (2012). Development of an educational brochure for premenopausal women following breast or gynecologic cancer treatment. Retrieved from https://nursing.vanderbilt.edu/images/dnp/scholarly/2012/2012Hodges.jpg

As you begin to shape your project, the key to the selection of your topic is to focus on what is already known and the relevance to *your* practice environment. It is not necessary to consider whether your chosen topic will benefit the entire population of people who share your interest. Rather, focus on selecting a topic that will meet your program requirements and address the needs of people in your neighborhood, agency, or specialty. The application of research in the field, wherever that may be, is the purpose of generating research. Sharing your experiences of how well research worked is what the individuals who completed the research are waiting to hear from you.

Practice-Based Scholarship

Practice-based scholarship comes in many forms. The definition of *practice-based scholarship* from the AACN is:

> The scholarship of practice has emerged in nursing as a critical component in the maintenance of clinical competency of faculty in a university setting and the advancement of clinical knowledge in the discipline (Norbeck & Taylor, 1998; Rudy et al., 1995; Wright, 1993). Practice scholarship encompasses all aspects of the delivery of nursing service where evidence of direct impact in solving health care problems or in defining the health problems of a community is presented. Competence in practice is the method by which knowledge in the profession is both advanced and applied. Practice roles for faculty in health care delivery systems may include direct caregiver, educator, consultant, and administrator (Brown et al., 1995; Norbeck & Taylor, 1998). (1999, "Scholarship of Practice")

The benefits of scholarship are viewed using internal measures of quality to the organization where the project will be conducted. Even though there has been confusion, there is increasing understanding of what a project is (Reid Ponte & Nicholas, 2015).

Terhaar and Sylvia (2016), in their study on assessing the quality of DNP projects, developed a list of the types of project completed at various universities. Their analysis of rigor in DNP projects demonstrates the scope, creativity, and importance of practice-based scholarship. A few topics you may consider include topics that highlight challenges and barriers to completing work on a day-to-day basis, including improvements to processes of patient care such as admission and discharge, patient and nurse educational resources, triage processes, and other follow-up for patients. With the current focus on decreasing admissions to the hospital in fewer than 30 days, selecting a topic relevant to any part of the discharge process, immediate follow-up, and coordination of care would be an asset to the patient, family, and organization. With a general goal of performance improvement, much can be done to assist practitioners, customers/clients, and the community to improve patient health. Selecting a topic from any one of these areas is appropriate. In later chapters the technique for refining the selected topic will be discussed.

Scholarly projects are shared through peer-review publications, presentations at conferences, through consultations, testimony, creating reports for specific audiences, grant applications, advanced certification, and many digital methods that include blogs, websites streaming video, and many more. Start a Google Scholar page as first step (Figure 2.1).

Discovery/Research Scholarship

Research, sometimes called *discovery scholarship*, is the creation of new knowledge through a systematic process of conducting empirical studies, and philosophical, clinical, policy, and regulatory-focused research (Boyer, 1990). Although many DNP programs began by requiring a research study, the trend is to follow the AACN guidelines discussed earlier and focus on a practice-based project. If you are considering a traditional research study, check with your advisor and university handbook for the specifics of what is required. As mentioned, the intent of this chapter is to use the SHARED model and to follow its steps to complete your DNP project.

A doctoral-level research study is often done as a replication or pilot study. Most DNP students must work within a very tight budget with limited time to collect and analyze data. Ask your advisor what university-level resources are available to assist with your study. In addition to a detailed procedure that describes university guidelines for proposing, conducting, and evaluating your study, there should be available statisticians, small amounts of money to pay for expenses related to conducting research, such as payment for office supplies, telephone costs, and similar expenses.

Here is an example of a small pilot study I conducted:

Atheists' Preferences for End-of-Life Care

In 2006, I conducted a small study to understand the preferences that atheists had for their end-of-life care (Smith-Stoner, 2007). After years of working in hospice, I knew that many hospice workers were very religious and numerous patients had expressed objections to nurses and others praying with them or trying to convert them to a religion. I was curious as to what beliefs atheists possessed about end-of-life care and wanted to know what we (in hospice) could do to support their beliefs more effectively.

After identifying the problem—the gap in care—the next step was to conduct a small study (it was very difficult to find a group to participate) to explore whether my clinical observations were accurate for a larger population than the patients I cared for in Southern California. After searching for groups of atheists, I found some who agreed to send a notice about the intended study to their members asking whether they would complete an online survey.

To obtain permission to conduct the study, I applied for permission from the university institutional review board (IRB). The process is straightforward but requires compliance with local and federal rules for the protection of participants. Research courses in your program will provide more information on how to conduct research than is possible include to here.

I collected the information, then analyzed, and published it about a year after first obtaining permission to do the study. My dissemination strategy at that time was very traditional: present the results at palliative care and other hospice-related conferences via a podium or poster presentation.

Although many academics and hospice clinicians found my article through library searches, a new population found the study through a single reference in Richard Dawkins's (the famous English advocate for secularism), bestselling book

The God Delusion. I received many inquiries from the press as a result. It was an interesting time for me to grow professionally as I navigated the general public's approval and disapproval of the study.

Since the study was first published, many clinicians have used this article in their literature reviews for other studies that inform the addition of knowledge to spiritual care for patients and their family. Walsh and McGoldrick's (2013) use is an example of practice translation. The authors applied the original research and incorporated it into their work with families that were bereaved. It was very satisfying to see a simple online study get disseminated beyond my own direct activities. The right topic has the potential to provide exposure for knowledgeable clinicians with a passion for the topic.

☐ How to Find Your Research/Practice Topics

To find a topic, reach others and listen to their needs, concerns, and hopes for the future. The list of potential practice topics is far longer than anyone can imagine. The challenge is to find a project that is important to the organization, interesting to investigate, and meeting the program guidelines. Strategic plans, professional practice initiatives, changes in reimbursement, quality data, patient satisfaction surveys, community health issues, threats to the health of children in schools, portions of the community, the health of community groups such as church members, the homeless, and other shelters are a few of the locations that can always use an evidence-based health-related service project.

FIGURE 2.1 **Smith-Stoner and Google Scholar.**

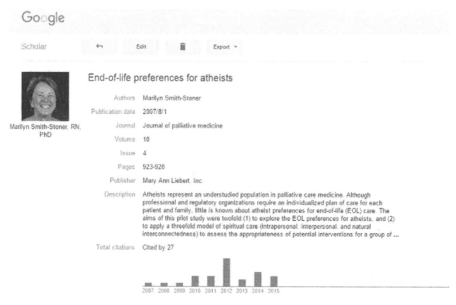

Traditional searches in your university online databases can determine whether there is enough existing evidence to provide for the translation into practice necessary for a DNP project. Google Scholar, along with your university library interface, makes this process simple. Setting up automated alerts in the online library databases and in Google helps ensure you stay up to date with new information as it is published or posted on the Internet. Begin by setting up your Google Scholar page and create alerts there. Check out the many YouTube videos (also owned by Google) to show you how.

Another example of research-to-practice topics is an integrative review. The absolute leader in integrative reviews is Cecelia Crawford, RN, DNP, of Kaiser Permanente in Southern California. For her culminating work in the DNP program at Western University, she investigated and devised a Collaborative Center for Integrative Reviews and Evidence Summaries (CCIRES) to create integrative reviews and evidence summaries (Crawford, 2012) to narrow the education–practice–research group. At the Southern California Kaiser Permanente website, you can find many of the integrative summaries she developed with others to help develop practice guidelines from her research. Dyan Summers, RN, DNP is a hero. She applied her education to be the first clinician to recognize the Zika virus in the United States (Piore, 2016).

☐ Preparing for a Study

You'll be taking entire courses that focus on research and evaluation. The information provided here offers a summary to help you understand the entire process of dissemination. All studies and projects involve collecting data in libraries, which is also called *research*. It helps to describe the first step as "collecting evidence" rather than "research." Then collecting prior literature is not confused with conducting a research study by others not familiar with your school's system of doing a capstone project.

As you collect evidence, organize that evidence into some type of meaningful format, a table of evidence is usually the suggested form preferred by universities. A traditional table of evidence is usually focused on research studies exclusively, so it is missing a lot of other types of evidence. Include regulations, professional practice statements, art, literature, and stories of current events that are shaping practice, such as medical errors, in the news in your table. You can also use applications, such as Zotero, to collect, organize, and retrieve evidence.

After identifying a gap or the significance of a patient care issue, construct a plan for collecting and analyzing evidence. Table 2.2 describes the difference between research and quality improvement (QI), primarily that QI is used internally in an organization, and research is meant to be used externally as well. Both will involve a process of being systematic and transparent in your work. However, the ultimate consumers of your work are nonacademic. Your QI, practice-based project focuses on the organization where the project is conducted. Others may want to replicate the same project and add to the body of knowledge, but the primary intention of the QI project is to use the information garnered internally.

TABLE 2.2 **Comparison of Research and Quality Improvement**

Research	Quality Improvement
Identifies a gap in practice Can also identify a process that works very effectively and wants to describe in detail to replicate Usually begins with a thorough review of existing literature Can incorporate a theoretical model Requires institutional review board approval for protection of participants in the form of a consent Use a hierarchy of research quality such as Johns Hopkins Rating Scale (Newhouse, Dearholt, Poe, Pugh, & White, 2005) Audience: entire research community	Identifies a gap in practice: structure, process, or outcome of care Can also identify a process that works very effectively and wants to describe in detail to replicate Begins with a review of the literature, consideration of regulations, financial imperatives, regulatory mandates, or other practice changes Conditions of admission may give a blanket permission for all people who receive care to have their records accessed for additional analysis Summarizes process through a logic model Can incorporate a theoretical model Audience: internal community
Quantitative: Uses multiple statistical analyses according to the types of data (nominal, ordinal, ratio, and interval) using specific methods; examples are inferential and noninferential statistics; the entire process is public and reported so that readers of reports can independently evaluate the trustworthiness of process and results	Uses a variety of statistics, depending on the level of analysis; in a single agency, data may focus more on descriptive statistics and compare differences between groups Data are collected as an internal matter of the agency and generally not shared publicly beyond general information to stakeholders about quality and customer satisfaction initiatives
Qualitative: Gathers holistic information using phenomenological, ethnographic, and other methods from small groups and analyzes transcripts of interviews (most common) according to various processes; the entire process is public and reported so that readers of reports can independently evaluate trustworthiness of process and results	Qualitative data usually focus on satisfaction due to recent changes in reimbursement related to value-added pricing and increased emphasis on pay for performance; satisfaction is focused on discharge surveys that are processed by third-party vendors and results are reported in themes
Mixed methods	Can involve a combination of patient, financial, or other data usually public and private; a common method used is Plan-Do-Study-Act

(continued)

TABLE 2.2 **Comparison of Research and Quality Improvement (*continued*)**

Research	Quality Improvement
Meant to be generalizable	Focused on only agency or service within that agency
Meant to be replicable	Meant for an agency, community, or specific system
Focused on specific populations	Focused on specific agency

☐ Review Board Approval

Activities that require approval of the IRB include giving people a survey and then publishing or otherwise reporting the results of the survey or manipulating anything that may cause mental or physical harm to another. Some organizations will see a survey as exempt from review, others will not. However, you are not authorized to determine whether a project is exempt from IRB approval, you must submit the application to the IRB and let its members determine that. There are also different levels of approval. A simple survey may take a couple of days to approve, so there is nothing to worry about as long as you have completed the application appropriately. When there is very little risk to the people completing the survey, the application is readily approved. Often this is called an "exempt" review, meaning it is exempt from the need for the entire committee to approve the study.

A typical kind of survey that may need to be reviewed is a test–retest survey done before and after a class is given. If you want to do a survey before and after the presentation of some type of intervention, to assess changes in attitude, skills, or other variables, there may be some issues with students. Students may have some risk in participating if you are going to identify the survey takers and compare results for each person (which is a good idea). The IRB would want to make sure the participants' scores would not be given to their supervisors, which may result in a punitive job action. That is the ethical protection of human participants in research.

☐ Quality Improvement

Continuous QI is the lifeblood of all health care. There are always problems that can be solved by ongoing inquiry into the root causes of an internal problem. One important difference between a research study and QI is that QI uses the products of research to improve the quality of care. Said another way, when an organization, unit, or stakeholder within an organization identifies a problem, the first step to finding a solution is to see what solutions have been found already in previous research. Instead of conducting a formal research study, members of a QI committee may translate existing information from one situation to another. There are times when an agency has no choice, because there is a lack of research on a wide range of practice issues. It is often necessary for advance practice nurses to begin with an internal study to assess local issues on a clinical issue before undertaking a formal study.

The QI plan to evaluate the effectiveness of the project is evaluated through measuring changes in outcomes. At the present time, patient satisfaction is one of the most common topics of QI projects as reimbursement is not tied, in part, to satisfaction scores. A QI project on noise reduction at one hospital may or may not be generalizable to other hospitals because there are many factors that can impact noise levels. As a result, before and after measurements of noise levels, patient and staff satisfaction can vary widely from agency to agency. There will be some type of statistical analysis in translational projects, but they are not designed to be generalizable beyond the agency sponsoring the work and usually do not need the rigorous process of research analysis. They also may not have the number or diversity of participants that are needed to utilize high-powered statistics and the issue under study may not be something that an agency wants to publicly disclose.

☐ Translational Research

Translational research is the newest form of generating nursing knowledge. As Grady (2010) stated:

> Translational research transforms scientific findings or discoveries from basic laboratory, clinical, or population studies into new clinical tools, processes, or applications. (p. 164)

Common translational projects will include planning, implementation, and evaluation of clinically significant projects by individuals or teams of individuals. The objective of the plan will be to focus on a change that impacts care outcomes in some way only at the clinician's agency. At the doctoral level, projects look at the local systems or population or community level, for example, reviewing data on patients who smoke or share a specific disease condition in a community. The project usually includes some type of intervention to improve the lives of individuals (the population in the city where the hospital is located). Although there are many gaps in the system of changing practice based on the best available evidence, the focus in this book is on best practices for informing professionals and lay people about evidence and to inspire a greater level of implementation of quality information by bring dissemination strategies into the 21st century. In order to make significant use of relevant evidence, all forms of dissemination, including social media, the arts, multimedia, and traditional broadcast methods, need access to the information in meaningful ways. That is the purpose of this book, to show advanced practice nurses that there are a multitude of ways to get your message out. And there is no time to waste, the lives of clinicians and patients depend on it.

☐ Conclusions

Understanding the differences between a research and practice-based project is essential to selecting your topic and planning you project. A full description of how to conduct a project can be found in many publications dedicated to the topic. While you are selecting your topic and confirming whether you are doing a research- or practice-based project, take note of where you are finding information. The location and type of information you find may provide you with some insight into the best dissemination methods. If you find yourself reading journals, then consider using a publication for dissemination. However, it is more likely that you are using a combination of web-based information, social media, video streaming, and other digital resources. As you continue to record your progress in your journal, be sure to add in contact and reference information so you can refer to it later. You will be discussing your project informally and formally during and after you complete your degree. Practice-based quality projects are very important for patient care at a single facility or system. The products of systematically collected data from rigorous research studies are the tools that clinicians use to restructure care beyond a single agency.

REFERENCES

American Association of Colleges of Nursing. (1999). Defining scholarship for the discipline of nursing. Retrieved from http://www.aacnnursing.org/News-Information/Position-Statements-White-Papers/Defining-Scholarship

American Association of Colleges of Nursing. (2015). The doctor of nursing practice: Current issues and clarifying recommendations. Retrieved from http://www.aacnnursing.org/Portals/42/DNP/DNP-Implementation.pdf?ver=2017-08-01-105830-517

Boyer, E. L. (1990). *Scholarship reconsidered: Priorities for the professoriate.* Princeton, NJ: Carnegie Foundation for the Advancement of Teaching.

Brown, S. A., Cohen, S. M., Kaeser, L., Leane, C. D., Littleton, L. Y., Otto, D. A., & Rickman, K. J. (1995). Nursing perspective on Boyer's scholarship paradigm. *Nurse Educator, 20*(5), 26–30.

Crawford, C. L. (2012). *Using a collaborative center for integrative reviews and evidence summaries to narrow the education-practice-research gap.* Retrieved from https://pqdtopen.proquest.com/doc/1346223204.html?FMT=ABS

Grady, P. (2010). What is translational research? *Nursing Outlook, 58,* 164–166. Retrieved from https://www.ninr.nih.gov/sites/www.ninr.nih.gov/files/NursingOutlookMay _June2010PAGTranslationalresearch.pdf

Newhouse, R., Dearholt, S., Poe, S., Pugh, L. C., White, K. (2005). The Johns Hopkins Nursing Evidence-Based Practice Rating Scale. Retrieved from http://www.mc .vanderbilt.edu/documents/CAPNAH/files/Mentoring/Section%206/JHNEDP %20Evidence%20Rating%20Scale.pdf

Norbeck, J. S., & Taylor, D. L. (1998). Faculty practice. In E. Sullivan (Ed.), *Creating nursing's future: Issues, opportunities and challenges.* St. Louis, MO: C. V. Mosby.

Piore, A. (2016, May 9). Nursing school doctorate graduate finds first case of Zika virus. *Columbia News.* Retrieved from http://news.columbia.edu/node/1116

Reid Ponte, P., & Nicholas, P. K. (2015). Addressing the confusion related to DNS, DNSc, and DSN degrees, with lessons for the nursing profession. *Journal of Nursing Scholarship, 47*(4), 347–353. doi:10.1111/jnu.12148

Rudy, E. B., Anderson, N. A., Dudjak, L., Robert, S. N., & Miller, R. A. (1995). Faculty practice: Creating a new culture. *Journal of Professional Nursing, 11*(2), 78–83.

Smith-Stoner, M. (2007). End-of-life preferences for atheists. *Journal of Palliative Medicine, 10*(4), 923–928. Retrieved from http://www.ncbi.nlm.nih.gov/pubmed/17803415

Terhaar, M. F., & Sylvia, M. (2016). Scholarly work products of the doctor of nursing practice: One approach to evaluating scholarship, rigour, impact and quality. *Journal of Clinical Nursing, 25*(1/2), 163–174. doi:10.1111/jocn.13113

Walsh, F., & McGoldrick, M. (2013). Bereavement: A family life cycle perspective. *Family Science, 4*(1), 20–27. doi:10.1080/19424620.2013.819228

Wright, D. J. (1993). Faculty practice: Criterion for academic advancement. *Nursing and Health Care, 14*(1), 18–21.

CHAPTER 3

Choosing Your Method of Sharing Your Project

Chapter Checklist

☑	Planning
☑	Exploring
☑	Experimenting
☑	Assessing what you know
☑	Common mistakes to avoid

☐ Planning

Sharing both the process and the product of your doctoral journey involves identifying the audience that most needs to learn about your work and its preferred method of taking in new information. Your work, your unique addition to nursing science, focuses on a specific issue and group of people. Men and women, people of all ages, follow characteristic patterns of consuming new information. Marketing science includes finding out how and where to share your work. A few important sites will help you decide how to best reach your audience, and careful planning will help you reach the maximum number of people who are waiting to hear about the information you have created (Table 3.1).

TABLE 3.1 **Determining the Preferred Method of Consuming News**

	Resource	Website
1	Pew Research Center	www.pewresearch.org
2	Brandwatch	www.brandwatch.com/blog/social-media-analytics-tools
3	Hootsuite	http://signup.hootsuite.com
4	Tweetmap	http://tweetmap.com

The recent Pew Research Center report, "How Americans Encounter, Recall and Act Upon Digital News," states that community news is most likely to be shared by a friend or family member who see it on social media (Mitchell, Gottfried, Schearer, & Lu, 2017). If your topic is focused locally, share it via an online community forum, such as a Facebook page, printed newspaper, radio, or cable channel. The Pew Research Center publishes an annual report on social media updates to use to help you understand the process of targeting your message. If you are planning a traditional publication, consider using a tool, such as Altmetric, to track views. You can also find out the most viewed articles in a year there. Reviewing the topics can help you define a topic, too.

☐ Exploring

As you form your dissemination strategy, identify multiple potential methods for presenting your project. Whatever you decide, keep in mind that you are going to produce something that is worthy of and reflects doctoral-level accomplishment. Here is a chance to break out of the traditional PowerPoint lecture and show your creative, scholarly best. Consider using a tiered approach to sharing your process and product using both professional and popular media. Think of the possibilities as a continuum of traditional publications in scholarly journals and presentations at a nursing conference all the way to artistic methods such as a play or art exhibit. In between are many digital possibilities such as websites, podcasts, videos, ebooks, or other digital material. The choice is yours, and you have the responsibility to ensure the method you choose is acceptable to your university and accessible to the population that needs your information. Exploring possibilities is inexpensive as most accounts are free or have a limited free access and paid version for users.

The four most popular social media resources in 2017 are Facebook, YouTube, Twitter, and LinkedIn. The most used social media platforms vary from year to year and as may change as new resources are developed. When beginning the process of exploration, you will find user profiles at each of the media websites and the social media accounts of the experts you are including in your review of the literature on your subject. You are likely to find many on Facebook, in a podcast (iTunes, Stitcher, Patreon, and others), blog (web search), and SlideShare or LinkedIn (both owned by Microsoft). Keep notes of the best practices expert users display in their own social media in your journal. Most of these sites have a free level of service as well as a paid version.

☐ Experimenting

Once you've found some social media tools you think might work, start experimenting. Twitter is a great place to start. Create an account with a descriptive name of the general topic of focus. If you want some inspiration, try the family of topics from the website in the United Kingdom called #WeCommunities (www .wecommunities.org). Even if the character limit increases, start with 140 characters and some images, and begin posting basic information. You may post or "tweet" about what you are reading. Create images using the free tool "Canva. com" to add some graphics to your posts.

As you are reading material for classes, consider posting important or meaningful quotes with reference information. By exploring and using the tools, you will gain skill in posting to the specific social media and develop the habit of reading, saving, sharing, and creating posts.

☐ Assessing What You Know

Much of this book is devoted to giving very specific directions on how to complete specific types of dissemination projects once your project is complete. At this point, while you are still working on a project, you can work smarter and not harder by making some general decisions about your dissemination method as early as possible. Table 3.2 describes some methods of dissemination that will provide a lasting legacy of your work and share your hard work with the most number of people who will benefit from it.

☐ Creating the Plan

Regardless of the method you choose to tell the world about your project, the process begins with a written paper that summarizes the project, timelines, and methods you have selected. This plan must first meet the requirements of your university and secondarily describe the specifics of the method in sufficient detail to obtain approval for your dissemination methods.

TABLE 3.2 **Methods of Sharing Work**

Title	Source
Oral—traditional	Presentation at professional conference
	Testimony at public hearing
	Expert witness at court hearing
	Teaching of all kinds
	One-person show
	Table reading of a script
Oral—virtual	Video Vlog
	Audio podcast
	Vine—6-second video
	Real-time video collaboration: Blab, Google Hangout, Periscope
	Screen capture instructional videos
	Television or radio interview
Text	Article for publication
	Article describing project: clinical innovation
	Article: lessons learned from going back for advanced degree
	Article: lessons learned for future students
	Article: lessons learned related to technology
	Article: lessons learned from work–life balance
	Article: lessons learned from transformational experience
	Article: letters to the editor
	White paper reports on health issues for specific groups
	Professional reports for specific groups
	Patient or staff education handouts
	Surveys or polls
	Policy or procedure
Text—virtual	Blog
	Polls—surveys
	Newsletters
	Articles for the public
	Social media: Facebook, Twitter, Reddit

Your plan will ultimately be transformed into any one of a variety of formats. Whether you choose a podcast, blog, or theater production, the basis of each is content on the subject.

Your journal will supplement your official documents throughout the process of completing your project, serving as a guide for your project completion. Keep notes about things to do, insights you have gained while researching, using social media, talking with experts or others, and names of resources available to you in your journal. The journal also documents your emerging expertise in the subject you have chosen. As you move closer to graduation, you may be asked to describe the process you used to develop your topic. The journal will be the best resource to track your thought process.

Maintain organization all along the way. Keep all your assignments in one place. Organize everything in your computer in file folders that can be easily searched. The file structure may be by class or by topic. If your program requires a portfolio at the end to document your process, well-organized files will be invaluable.

The "best of the best" work will be included in the portfolio as one type of presentation of your best ideas on your topic to share with your faculty and other students. Ideally, your portfolio will be presented to peers and the community, too, via digital methods.

☐ Avoid These Common Mistakes

Using an Assignment "as is" as a Submission

In important ways, your project will make life better for the people you identified. Unless other clinicians know what you've found, very few people will benefit from your hard work. Therefore, many programs require submission of a final paper for the purpose of publication.

To share your work with others, it must appear outside the walls of your school. An assignment is usually shared with your peers, family, and faculty. They have looked at the paper/assignment with an eye toward course compliance, not the eyes of persons who will actually use the information. It is entirely likely that your faculty advisor is not an expert in your topic. Committee members and the chair may have varying degrees of content expertise; however, they are likely to understand the procedures to complete doctoral-level work at your university.

If you are required to submit an article for publication, it must conform to the author guidelines of the journal. You will find the guidelines on the journal website. It is likely that the guidelines will require you to edit your article. To have your article considered, the format, length, headers, referencing, and other style attributes must follow the guidelines. The editor will work with you when your ideas meet the focus of the journal. Don't hesitate to call the editor or send an email query in advance of submission. Editors are often educators and their skill will turn your first submission into a publication when you plan carefully and collaborate with them.

☐ Take Every Opportunity to Present Your Work

Practice makes perfect. Seek out ways to present your work, even when your ideas are just starting to form. Find people who are affected by your topic or are connected in some way. The presentations may be done in churches, community groups, TV, radio, and blogs. Invite comments, critique, and feedback wherever you go.

If you are going to use a method, such as a blog or other web-based methods, include a strategy for responding to feedback as you are preparing your dissemination strategy. If you are placing something on the Internet, you can choose to enable or disable the comments section on a blog or other website where a video is posted. Each strategy will have a unique set of considerations for obtaining feedback.

If you appear on a TV or radio station, make sure to read comments on social media about the presentation. You can collect email addresses of people who attend your presentations or read your comments so you can let them know when updates are available. What is most important to others is that you are authentic and honest in your presentation. When you don't know something, say so. As a student, people will understand you are on a journey. Don't get ahead of yourself in the process.

When you are giving a public presentation, you can ask the organizer of the event for a copy of the program evaluation comments if they are not shared with you automatically. You may even ask to have your own evaluation completed if desired. If you post something on the Internet, you can measure its effectiveness and interest by looking at analytics, which are easy to obtain. Simple measures are the number of shares, comments, and links made to the material. More on each method is described in Unit IV. Keep all the evaluations to document your evolution in the program.

Small Audiences Have a Big Benefit

Irrespective of how small the audience, seek out opportunities to give a presentation to new groups that do not know your subject or you. The feedback from people who do not know you is invaluable. The feedback from people you are related to, have intimate relations with, or evaluate at work, can have serious limitations. Find impartial interested people to give you feedback every chance you get; your project will be better for it. In addition, you will also be developing the presentation skills you will need for your final presentation of the capstone project.

Look particularly for feedback if you are sharing your project via artistic methods such as poetry, a theater production, or video. Each of these methods has its own developmental process that is available to you. You may need to start as an intern or volunteer with an organization that is involved in the medium you are interested in to gain basic skills. Every moment spent developing basic skills in the area you want to use to disseminate your work is well worth the time and can probably be counted as part of your community volunteer hours, which are a requirement of DNP programs.

TABLE 3.3 Mobile Applications to Help Organize Files

	Application	Source
1	Evernote	http://evernote.com
2	Notability	www.gingerlabs.com
3	Google Drive	http://drive.google.com
4	Grammarly	https://app.grammarly.com
5	Microsoft One Drive	https://onedrive.live.com/about/en-us
6	Dropbox (many others)	http://dropbox.com

Remaining Current

To have a well-developed paper or script that reflects your work, you will need to maintain a current table of evidence. You will learn how to create a table of evidence in a research class. However, with each class you take, you will be adding valuable resources such as regulations, professional standards, clinical guidelines, ethics case studies, and other professional information. All of these references should be noted in a table of evidence, which will save a lot of time when you are ready to create your dissemination product.

Consider using mobile apps, such as Evernote or Noteability, to organize your files, including documents, pdfs, photographs, and audio and video files. You will then be able to easily retrieve files as you need them. Table 3.3 lists applications that can assist you in organizing all types of files. They are all free or offer a limited version that is free. Each works on all operating systems.

☐ Oral Presentations

Check your student handbook and ask your advisor about the types of presentations you must make to demonstrate you have achieved the program objectives. Whatever type you give, make it your best effort and incorporate doctoral-level skills and content into your presentation. Make it memorable for the people who consume the material. It won't cover your entire education, you will be selecting significant findings from your work to fit the interests of the audience and constraints of the platform you select. For example, a typical conference presentation lasts 15 to 30 minutes. Make each second count by being prepared, enthusiastic, and look amazing. You and your insight will make the presentation memorable, not the PowerPoint slides. There is no substitute for preparing a presentation that fits the audience, rather than using a set of slides done for a class project. Remember that less is more when giving a presentation. Study what makes a great presentation!

The Science of Public Speaking

There are two parts to a great presentation. First, to consider are the qualities of the presenter. Second, is the content. Spend time developing your presentation skills so people will want to hear about your work. Even when you are giving a presentation in class, a generally safe area, explore new ways of presenting, new techniques and using new technologies, such as interactive polling, while you are describing your project. Take the assessment in Figure 3.1 to see what your level of public-speaking skill is. If you need help, you will find many resources in this text to help you.

Self-assess your comfort with public speaking, and then start to improve your oral presentation skills. The best presentations tell a compelling story. They are created, practiced, modified, and continuously improved. No one else can deliver *your* presentation (Table 3.4).

TED Talks as the Gold Standard

In 1984, Richard Saul Wurman launched the phenomenon called *technology, entertainment and design (TED)*, which was initially unsuccessful. Six years later he tried again and the rest is history. Year by year, the TED movement has grown from an annual single conference in Monterey, California, to a wide array of TED events held all over the world. A TED presentation is short, dynamic, concise, and well rehearsed. Presenters don't read from notes, they make eye contact with a few people in the audience and tell a story that illustrates the broader principle (Anderson, 2013). They leave the audience wanting more. Modeling a TED-style presentation is an appropriate format for a traditional in-person oral or recorded presentation. The time limitations are roughly equal to a scholarly presentation at nursing conference. You can shake things up at a traditional nursing conference by producing one PowerPoint slide with a great image and your contact information and follow that with a dynamic, well-rehearsed presentation the audience will never forget.

The top 10 TED presentations (at the time of this writing; see https://www.ted.com/playlists/171/the_most_popular_talks_of_all):

1. Do schools kill creativity? Ken Robinson
2. Your body language shapes who you are, Amy Cuddy
3. How great leaders inspire action, Simon Sinek
4. The power of vulnerability, Brené Brown
5. My stroke of insight, Jill Bolte Brown
6. The thrilling potential of SixthSense technology, Pranav Mistry
7. 10 things you didn't know about orgasm, Mary Roach
8. Why we do what we do, Tony Robbins
9. The puzzle of motivation, Dan Pink
10. Underwater astonishments, David Gallo

The topics on this list are generic and of potential interest to everyone. Your topic may be one that has a universal appeal. But it is more likely to have a specialized focus. The principles of TED talks work. Every time you get in front of a group of people, however you do it, is an opportunity to change someone's life.

FIGURE 3.1 **Assessment for oral presentations.**

1	My greatest strength was:	
2	My second greatest strength was:	
3	My third greatest strength was:	
4	The primary method of presentation:	
	a Told a story that is as much personal as scientific	
	b Involved the audience in some way	
	c Included time for questions and answers	
	d Used PowerPoint slides	
5	What feelings were projected?	
	a I project confidence	
	b I looked like a deer in headlights	
	c I conveyed stage fright	
	d I was barely able to get my thoughts out	
6	Quality of posture	
	a Stood straight and tall or sat with a flat back	
	b Posture varied from beginning to end of interview/presentation	
	c Stood in one place	
	d Cowered /leaned behind the podium	
7	Where are your eyes pointed?	
	a Straight at the audience or interviewer	
	b Varied from direct eye contact to looking at the floor	

(*continued*)

FIGURE 3.1 **Assessment for oral presentations.** (*continued*)

	c	Looked at slides or notes over half the time	
	d	Looked at a few friendly faces in the front row	
8		What were you wearing?	
	a	Professional dress	
	b	Well-prepared scrubs or uniform	
	c	Whatever I was wearing that day	
	d	Street clothes	
9		Makeup and hair	
	a	Recent haircut and subtle makeup	
	b	Washed my hair the night before and wore my usual makeup	
	c	Pinned my hair back and wet my lips before the interview/presentation started	
	d	It depends on how much time I have before I leave the house	
10		Content of presentation	
	a	Clear, concise, and delivered within the time frame given	
	b	Stayed mostly on track or went over the time limit	
	c	Followed prepared presentations from publishers and others	
11		Body language	
	a	My body conveyed an open and enthusiastic presence	
	b	I generally kept my hands and feet under control	
	c	I could not seem to figure out how to stand/sit or what to do with my hands	
	d	My hands looked like airplanes in a dogfight	
12		Describe how the audience reacted to the presentation	

As you progress through your program, incorporate TED-style talks into your ongoing evidence presentations. You will find world-class researchers, thought leaders, and influencers giving TED talks. You may be able to have a direct communication with the individual expert through the many TED channels of communication, especially blogs, podcasts, and Twitter.

Great public presentations have a degree of authenticity and vulnerability. If you are a baby boomer, you will never forget the role the Monica Lewinsky extramarital affair had on the Clinton presidency. She gave an amazing TED talk in 2015 on shame and the role of shame in society (www.ted.com/talks/monica_lewinsky_the_price_of_shame/transcript?language=en).

Commencement and Specialized Speeches

Commencement and other specialized speeches can also teach what makes a great presentation. These are longer than the typical 15-minute professional scholarly presentation. Watch some of presentations suggested in this chapter and find some that resonate with you. Work on a few of the skills at a time. Little by little you will be able to deliver the same time of presentation. Links to the following presentations are excellent examples of speeches:

Steve Jobs, Commencement at Stanford, 2005. www.youtube.com/watch?v=D1R-jKKp3NA

Randy Pausch, Last lecture at Carnegie Melon, 2007. www.youtube.com/watch?v=ji5_MqicxSo

Barack Obama, Audacity of hope, 2004. www.youtube.com/watch?v=eWynt87PaJ0

Expert Testimony

A popular specialty for advanced practice nurses is legal consulting and expert testimony. Although becoming a legal nurse consultant requires an entire course of study, there are ways for you to present testimony on a single subject to demonstrate your expertise as part of a capstone project. When your project focuses on a change in public policy, your expertise will benefit the public debate.

Throughout your program, you will have various assignments that will enable you to investigate the sources of problems in health care systems. You could be talking to elected and other government officials in order to see a policy change. As you progress through your program, you are developing a unique level of expertise. When you start talking to others, you may be asked to testify at public hearings. You can also seek out opportunities to testify or present your ideas on public policy in local, state, regional, and federal issues. Take every opportunity you can to call, write, and visit elected officials, regulators such as your state's board of registered nursing, professional nursing organizations, and public advocacy organizations. They are waiting to hear from a skilled and educated nurse who is passionate about the same topic they care about.

Teaching

Nursing is synonymous with teaching. Whether you are going to teach patients, clinicians, members of the community, or students at a university, you will find

TABLE 3.4 **Sources for Enhancing Presentations**

Title	Source
Oral—traditional	TED Talks—view any TED talk
	Sinek, S. (2013). *Read how to deliver a TED talk: Secrets of the world's most inspiring presentations.* New York, NY: McGraw-Hill
	PODCAST iTunes: "The Public Speaker's Quick and Dirty Tips for Improving Your Communication Skills" Lisa B. Marshal
	Marshal, L. (2013). *Smart talk: The public speaker's guide to success in every situation.* New York, NY: St. Martin's Griffin
	Toastmaster's Club (www.toastmasters.org): This organization builds confidence and skill in public speaking
	Public Speaking Blog: Ginger Public Speaking www.gingerpublicspeaking.com/blog
Text	
Script-writing tips	www.movieoutline.com/screenwriting-resources.html
WikiHow script writing	www.wikihow.com/Write-a-Script
Video	
Animoto	https://animoto.com
iMovie	www.apple.com/mac/imovie
MovieMaker	http://windows.microsoft.com/en-us/windows/movie-maker
Audio Podcast	
Audacity	http://theaudacitytopodcast.com/tap060-how-to-record-and-edit-a-podcast-with-audacity
Wiki How podcasts	www.wikihow.com/Start-Your-Own-Podcast
Virtual Text	
Blog	http://snip.ly/dTLR#www.wikihow.com/Be-a-Good-Blogger
Polls/surveys	Poll Everywhere: www.polleverywhere.com SurveyMonkey: www.surveymonkey.com

that there are many tools to use to augment teaching. Like all presentations, a lesson can be made ineffective by an overdose of trivia and words. The most successful teachers are highly interactive and tuned in to the needs of their students, whoever they are.

No matter how well someone knows a topic, preparation is necessary. Preparing backup materials to highlight *only* the most significant components of the topic is necessary. If you are asked about something beyond your scope, tell the questioner that. Be honest about your limitations. Every project has limitations.

Your enthusiasm is the key to getting others enthusiastic about your work. Using selective stories to tell others about the problem, the activities you completed, and what happened as a result of your work can inspire other clinicians to address an important issue, help a patient to change a bad habit, or assist policy makers to pass new legislation. A great example of changing a law in California came from a young woman with brain cancer. Brittany Maynard (http://thebrittanyfund .org) volunteered to become the face for medical aid in dying (physician-assisted suicide). Through sharing her very private story of terminal cancer, she was able to be a key factor in passing the End of Life Option Act.

As of June 2016, Californians who are terminally ill can choose to end their lives with the assistance of a prescription that will provide for a comfortable last breath (www.compassionandchoices.org). Although physician-assisted suicide, as it was called, has been legal in other states and there is an impressive body of research on the topic, it was not statistics that made the difference for Governor Jerry Brown to sign the legislation into law. Rather, it was the face of a young woman who felt she was powerless against her terminal cancer that inspired many to support this controversial legislation. The authenticity and honesty in the face of adversity that Brittany Maynard display, ed moved many in ways that were not thought possible before she shared her story.

☐ Top Mistakes Students Make in Learning Something New

As you start to determine what new and exciting method you will incorporate into your dissemination strategy, you will need to make some plans to manage your time effectively. You must follow the required guidelines of the organization sponsoring the dissemination presentation. Review this list of common mistakes and anticipate what you will do if you are tempted to do any of the following:

1. When you meet an obstacle, instead of working through it, you change your topic.
2. When learning to use a new technology, you do not allow enough time to master the technology before using it. This usually occurs through selecting sophisticated technology.
3. Assume your child is knowledgeable about your technical needs. However good the relationship is, it doesn't seem to work in this context.
4. Go for cheesy or amateurish skits instead of quality in presentation material.

5. Do not practice using the technology in the place the presentation will be made in advance.
6. Do not practice the presentation enough to know it by heart.
7. Do not follow the presentation guidelines, usually extending past the time allotment.
8. Use too many PowerPoint slides.
9. You try to "wing it."

☐ Conclusions

Presenting your material is the icing on your capstone cake. Regardless of how you feel about your project at the end of your program, others want to know what you did and how it relates to them. In other words, it matters what you have done. Letting others know about it and leaving a legacy for others to "follow in your footsteps" helps improve the lives of patients and their families. Presenting your project is the first substantial work you will do that demonstrates you are doctorally prepared and how hard you worked to obtain the degree. Let others celebrate and benefit from your success.

REFERENCES

Anderson, C. (2013). Giving a killer presentation. Retrieved from http://blog.ted.com/chris-anderson-shares-his-tips-for-giving-a-killer-presentation

Mitchell, A., Gottfried, J., Schearer, E., & Lu, K. (2017). How Americans encounter, recall and act upon digital news. Retrieved from http://www.journalism.org/2017/02/09/how-americans-encounter-recall-and-act-upon-digital-news

CHAPTER 4

Determining the Unique Contribution to Health Care

☐ Chapter Checklist

☑	"S" is selecting the subject and tool in the SHARED model.
☑	Practice inquiry projects: How do the results of your project change the lives of people touched by your project?
☑	Are there any "sacred cows" in the profession that can be eliminated because of your project?
☑	Does your project improve satisfaction of employees, patients, or consumers?
☑	Does your project improve the understanding of a complex problem?
☑	What are the priority areas of your nursing specialty organization?
☑	How does your project relate to *Healthy People 2020*?
☑	In what ways can your project support the mission, vision, and values of your organization?
☑	What accreditation standards are related to your topic?
☑	What health care concerns relate to your community?
☑	How are vulnerable populations in your community affected by health concerns?

☑	Can you transform your project related to illness to have a wellness or prevention focus?
☑	As a result, of your project, will practice, policies, or procedures change?
☑	How to use theoretical frameworks and other methods to shape your project.

☐ "S"=Select

A graduate project is meant to change something: However focused and "small" it may look to you, it is meant to improve the lives of people in your community, patients in your hospital, clients served by agencies in your community, or your colleagues, among many other possibilities. It is common that a topic will expand the knowledge and understanding of a population not previously addressed in the literature. Examples of expanding the understanding of the health needs means taking "bench to bedside to curbside" (Riner, 2015, p. 201). Taking a subject to the curbside, here, this means the community, could include projects with people who may be veterans; are gay, lesbian, bisexual, transgender (LGBT); or perhaps aging elderly caregivers caring for parents who are centenarians. Other topics include people with low literacy, learning disabilities, and sensory impairment. Think about your expertise and determine whether you could care for someone throughout the life span, someone with autism, a non-English speaker, or an individual who is transgender, a refugee, or a foster child. By applying your existing expertise to a new population, you are changing nursing practice and enhancing nursing science.

Throughout your course of study, you read, reflect, analyze, and report on a wide variety of important issues, research methodologies, health care regulations, and political controversies. As a result, you have a unique perspective based on the combined evidence collected, your knowledge, experience, and personal preferences. It is up to you to sculpt a very exciting process and to integrate your interests into your university requirements. This unique perspective, along with your analysis that incorporates evidence, contradictory information, discussion of gaps in science and suggestions for future areas of research, is what makes your project a unique practice inquiry.

Practice Inquiry Projects

"Practice inquiry" (Riner, 2015) is "an ongoing, systematic investigation of questions about nursing therapeutics and clinical phenomena with the intent to appraise and translate all forms of 'best evidence' to practice, and to evaluate the translational impact on the quality of health care and health outcomes." As you collect evidence, you will need a clear system for tracking what the project is and the progress you are making toward completion.

☐ Types of Projects

Shaking Up the Status Quo

Selecting your project can start with a courageous look at the status quo. Find that topic, that place in health care where you have ideas, you have insight into the dynamic system surrounding the systems involved with the potential practice change and focus there. Some suggestions include implementing a new health care form for people being discharge from some correctional facilities, implement the use of a stress-reduction mobile application for nursing staff on a unit, or create visual-cue campaign to increase compliance with hand hygiene.

The general types of projects are translational research, program evaluation, practice change, quality improvement, and translating evidence into practice. Each of these types of projects, done in different locations or in specific units in the hospital or populations, may lead to a unique contribution to nursing science.

Improving Satisfaction of Employees, Patients, or Consumers

Since the implementation of the Affordable Care Act and value- based payment (www.cms.gov/medicare/medicare-fee-for-service-payment/physicianfeedback program/valuebasedpaymentmodifier.html), patient satisfaction has evolved to be a key competitive metric as well as a financial factor. Efforts to ensure patients and their families have a positive feeling toward the care they received are now tied to payment (Kulkarni, 2016). Expanding existing research to new areas can provide care and comfort to patients and their families and enhance the financial stability of your agency. An example of this type of project could relate to the existing body of literature on the impact of photographs at a patient's bedside (Andersson, Hall-Lord, Wilde-Larsson, & Persenius, 2013). In Ansersson et al.'s study, nurses engaged in communication with patients and their family members when a photograph of the patient was placed at the bedside. There are a limitless number of variations to use to translate this type of practice change project. Perhaps the patient undergoing a hip replacement would benefit from taking a photo of him- or herself engaged in a favorite activity into surgery. Modifications on this theme can apply to many settings and types of patients.

Regardless of the type of project undertaken, it is important to follow a rigorous, transparent, and systematic process that builds on existing knowledge related to the purpose of your project. In order to facilitate application of the knowledge and insight you develop, it is important for future potential users to replicate the project.

Improve the Understanding of a Complex Problem

There are a whole host of "edutainment" programs that take very complex subjects and help others understand them. The most notable are the various types of "technology, education and design" (TED) talks. Since 1984, TED talks have evolved to be a force to be studied. All of the 18-minute videos are freely available online. TED conferences are held all over the world and present topics involved in the patient and health care professional experience. There are TED talks on dying, living longer, antibiotics, and cancer research, among many others. You can be inspired by the work of other nurses who have given TED talks or find the perfect idea for your own project through a search of their website (Ted.com).

Priority Areas of Your Nursing Specialty Organization

Each nursing and specialty organization has a list of its priority or research topics. A review of the websites of organizations related to your practice will reveal an important set of practice areas that are a focus of their research, education, and policy initiatives. If you are not already a member of your nursing practice professional association, as a student it is a good time to become a member of your professional association so that you can access the resources of the organization. Benefits typically include publications, conferences, possible mentors, and maybe scholarships. Once you graduate, you can become a leader through mentoring others, presenting at conferences, and using the SHARED model to let others know about your expertise. The Hospice and Palliative Nurses Association has a 3-year agenda on their website (http://hpna.advancingexpertcare.org/wp-content/uploads/2015/01/2015-2018-HPNA-Research-Agenda.pdf). Among many priority areas of interest are the management of dyspnea and fatigue. The Emergency Nurses Association has published priorities that include crowding/boarding, workplace violence, and care of psychiatric patients. Another type of initiative is the Nurses On Boards Coalition (2017). This coalition of nursing organizations has a goal of 10,000 nurses on board by 2020. Here is an established organization that may be able to help you with a public policy or advocacy-focused project and you may end up influencing others by being on a board.

Healthy People 2020

The Healthy People 2020 initiative is a significant project with a mission for a society in which all people live long, healthy lives (U.S. Department of Health and Human Services, 2014). Within its website are interactive tools with data, webinar access, and many more sources of potential practice-change topics. Leading health indicators that are part of the national Healthy People 2020 endeavor include topics on maternal–child health, nutrition and obesity, mental health and injury prevention, among many others.

Mission, Vision, and Values of Your Organization

Another source of inspiration for a practice-change project can be the website of your employer. Looking beyond the initiative on your own unit, check out what other health-related programs are part of your hospital or agency. There may be projects of interest in primary care, home services, community education, or marketing that are interesting to you and meet the objectives of your doctoral program.

Health Care Concerns in Your Community

In addition to national and state initiatives, there are organizations that track the health needs of specific areas. The Health Assessment and Research for Communities (HARC; 2017) in Southern California is one such resource for discovering the health care needs of people in your region—do an Internet search with your region's name and health care resources. A hub of resources is available from the Rural Health Initiative Hub (www.ruralhealthinfo.org). This hub is specifically related to care and issues related to people who live in rural areas of the United States. If your agency serves a large area, consider expanding an existing project to an emerging or part of the service area without an established health care infrastructure. Another twist is to look at how health care services are affected after a natural disaster in any part of your surrounding area. Or consider a review of the compliance with established vaccination schedules throughout populations in a region. Other creative ideas can be found at the University of Utah, in the report "Cultivating Collaboration" (2012).

Vulnerable Populations

Vulnerable populations refers to individuals who are economically disadvantaged, members of minorities, and others with limited access to health care. Those who are vulnerable include the homeless, the mentally ill, the poor, refugees, and immigrants. They can also be people who work fulltime or have more than one job but lack health insurance.

Care of people in a community without access to health care versus those who can afford to obtain their medication, access primary care, and follow-up care as required for their chronic health care conditions looks very different. Disparities are exacerbated when there is a language barrier. A practice project focused on non–English-speaking patients who have chronic conditions may be a significant contribution to the people in your community.

From Illness to Wellness

There are many types of projects that can be done with a focus on working upstream along the illness continuum. A critical care specialist can focus on home care. A mother–baby nurse can work in a community health center or high school child-care center.

Although each student's project has unique characteristics, the project should be significant enough that colleagues and other facilities share in the challenges addressed.

Many universities have included a list of DNP projects on their website. In 2015, Richardson analyzed the public availability of capstone project information on websites (Richardson, 2015). She determined there were many lists of projects available. Complete a comprehensive web search when you are ready to identify a topic. The possible types of topics are listed in Table 4.1. Examples of specific DNP project repositories are listed in Table 4.2.

TABLE 4.1 **Summary of DNP Practitioner Focus of Projects**

Translational science	Association of Clinical and Translational Science: www.actscience.org
Program evaluation	Formal evaluation of programs such as continuing education, internships, and residencies
Practice change (improvement) programs	Implementation of bench-to-beside projects that apply findings from research studies to patient care
Quality improvement	Continuous process of assessment and evaluation of care unique to an organization; may or may not be generalizable to others

TABLE 4.2 **Examples of Practice Inquiry Projects Databases**

	University	Resource
1	University of Missouri	List of projects: http://nursing.missouri .edu/academic-programs/dnp/doctor -nursing-practice-program-projects
2	Ohio State University	Examples of projects
3	University of Washington	List of references

☐ Highlighting the Unique Aspects of a Project

Whether you have already completed your project or are just beginning to plan it, your goals and objectives are the key to presenting your expertise and insight. The goals and objectives of the project describe what you are investigating, the population/subject under review, and variables that are of particular interest. After completing the first phase of the literature review on the topic, organize the evidence (articles, websites, applications, multimedia, social media posts, and visual content) so that it is easily retrievable.

☐ Careful Record Keeping

By maintaining a journal of your activities, thoughts, and reflections, it will be easier to describe the transformation of your thoughts and attitudes throughout the project. By having a chronological written, video, or other type of journal, you'll be able to demonstrate to others how your thinking changed from initially organizing the project through the evaluation. Having this rich source of your own insight "brands" the project to you and only you (see Table 4.2).

As your project progresses, the references will be organized according to the formatting guidelines of the university. Continually update the collection of evidence throughout your participation in the program. Continuously evaluating the sources used, while eliminating lower quality references, ensures your project meets the highest standards of academic excellence.

☐ Other Sources of Uniqueness

There is an endless combination of project attributes that define your project as significant and unique. The use of a specific theoretical framework, a way of knowing, a population, location, and many other variables contribute to the importance of your project. A comprehensive list of variables for capstone project that could make yours unique is available in Exhibit 4.1

EXHIBIT 4.1 **List of Concepts to Distinguish Project**

1. Theoretical framework
   a. Nursing theory
   b. Quality: Plan-Do-Act
   c. Organizational: Appreciative inquiry
2. Population
3. Context
4. Organization
5. Perspective—stakeholder
   a. Administration
   b. Patient/client
   c. Staff
   d. Public
   e. Policy makers
6. Ways of knowing
   a. Empirical
   b. Aesthetic
   c. Ethical
   d. Personal
7. Metaphors
8. Humor

☐ Theoretical Frameworks

There are many types of theoretical frameworks that can be used to help you structure your project. There are nursing theories and models, educational frameworks, quality improvement processes, and research methods that assist you in defining the problem or gap in knowledge to address the issue. Theoretical frameworks help view a problem or situation holistically. Some universities require use of a specific theory or model. In many cases, more than one framework will be used to structure the project and evaluate the results.

Ways of Knowing

Carper (1978) defined four patterns—empirical, aesthetic, ethical, and personal—of knowing as fundamental to understanding nursing. Including one or more ways of knowing helps to distinguish your projects (Figures 4.1 and 4.2).

☐ Review of Types of DNP Projects

Translational Science

Translational research transforms research findings from highly technical language to more usable applications of science for use in patient and other care. Often referred to as "bench to bedside," many DNP projects will be translational in nature.

FIGURE 4.1 **Ways of knowing.**

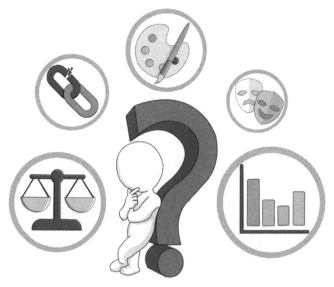

Holistic Method of Collecting Evidence for Nursing Practice

Program Evaluation

A common aspect of program evaluation is to measure the effectiveness of education programs such as continuing education for nurses. As part of all accreditation standards, program evaluation is an ongoing process in nursing education programs. In clinical areas, program evaluation of continuing education is best measured by outcomes, such as errors, injuries, and satisfaction, rather than the number of participants or course type and range of topics (American Nurses Credentialing Center, 2014).

Practice Change

Practice changes are developed and conducted in the clinical environment. Types of practice change evaluation projects can include practice guidelines from governmental or professional organizations and changes in staffing mix such as adding new specialties like advanced practice nurses.

☐ Quality Improvement

Quality-improvement studies are designed to improve the care in a single organization or system. The results of studies don't usually obtain institutional review as many are exempt from review. However, if you are planning on disseminating information from such a study, it is essential that you notify the public relations officer and review board to let them know there will be a publication that mentions the name of the organization in the author affiliation information.

Your Writing Style

Each person has a unique writing style. Your style can include use of specific terms, metaphors, humor, colors, inclusion activities, images, and many other aspects of presentation (Table 4.3). Developing your own style takes time. Consistently work on developing metaphors that are meaningful to you and relevant to your project. Going back to Aristotle,the idea existed that: *The greatest thing by far is to be a master of metaphor.*

Some examples of metaphors include:

- From my doctoral program at the California Institute of Integral Studies: *"PhD Students are midwives of Social Change"*
- Nurses are part jugglers, part artists, and part healers

Metaphors can be emphasized by combining the words with images from Unsplash.com or MorgueFile.com for copyright-free resources with free images. See the comprehensive list of image sources in Appendix 2.

FIGURE 4.2 **Example of a reference outline for a capstone project.**

Goal 1

Purpose 1

Theoretical model

Problem

Population

Context

Organization

Stakeholder perspective

Epistemology: Ways of knowing (Carper, 1978)

Carper, B.(1978),Fundamental ways of knowing in nursing. Advances in Nursing Science,1(1), 13–24. Retrieved from http://journals.lww.com/advancesinnursingscience/ Citation/1978/10000/Fundamental_Patterns_of_Knowing_in_Nursing_.4.aspx"-MPS"

TABLE 4.3 **Resources for Establishing a Unique Style**

Metaphors	
Healing story alliance	http://healingstory.org/publications/diving-in-the-moon-journal-2014/the-mystery-and-magic-of-metaphor/?doing_wp_cron=1503401443.9691948890686035156250
Finding and creating a metaphor	http://bit.ly/2bofBVu
Introducing metaphors through poetry	https://edsitement.neh.gov/lesson-plan/introducing-metaphors-through-poetry
Colors	
Psychological properties of colors	www.colour-affects.co.uk/psychological-properties-of-colours
Understanding the meaning of colors in color psychology	www.empower-yourself-with-color-psychology.com/meaning-of-colors.html
Humor	
The only two ways to tell a joke in presentations	www.forbes.com/sites/jerryweissman/2015/01/26/the-only-two-ways-to-tell-a-joke/#46f65a0f493f
How to be funny without telling a joke	www.wikihow.com/Be-Funny-Without-Telling-Jokes
Have them "rolling in the aisles" not "rolling their eyes"; how to tell jokes in a business presentation	www.speaklikeapro.co.uk/Jokes.htm
Taking your own photographs	
Photo gallery: How to take camera-phone pictures	www.nationalgeographic.com/photography/photo-tips/camera-phone-photos/#/fountain-portrait-england_23020_600x450.jpg
Take better smartphone photos with these 15 tips	www.usatoday.com/story/tech/columnist/saltzman/2014/06/07/how-to-take-better-smartphone-photos/9904509
Digital photography school	http://digital-photography-school.com/14-ways-to-significantly-improve-your-photography-today

(continued)

TABLE 4.3 **Resources for Establishing a Unique Style (*continued*)**

	Graphic design
Photography/Graphics	www.nationalgeographic.com/photography/photo-tips/camera-phone-photos/#/fountain-portrait-england_23020_600x450.jpg
Graphics design basics	www.thoughtco.com/what-is-graphic-design-1697521

TABLE 4.4 **Interactive Teaching Activities**

	Title	Source
1	Nurse author Michele Deck is considered a leader in interactive teaching	http://micheledeck.com/
2	Interactive techniques	www.fctl.ucf.edu/TeachingAndLearning Resources/CourseDesign/Assessment/content/101_Tips.pdf
3	Interactive presentations	www.crazyegg.com/blog/online -presentation-tools
4	*Forbes* magazine	www.forbes.com/sites/work-in-progress/2014/01/28/five-easy-tricks-to-make -your-presentation-interactive/#286d64192586
5	Collection of resources for 2016	www.customshow.com/best-powerpoint -alternatives-presentation-programs

Presentation Style

You can develop a presentation style that is uniquely yours. When people familiar with your work see the first images of your presentation, they will know it is yours. First and foremost do that by using consistent colors, fonts, and images.

Second, be known as someone who is as interested in what others haved to say as what you have to say. Find the best method of including the audience from start to finish during your presentation. Mobile applications like polleverywhere. com work well for that. Table 4.4 has a list of my selection of the best interactive activities.

☐ Conclusions

Your work product is unique as you are. Only you could have put the pieces together in the way you have. Always be clear about your focus and stay on track with the original purpose. Work through obstacles as they arise. There are always obstacles to important work. The point is to have confidence in what you are doing and not be deterred by others.

REFERENCES

American Nurses Credentialing Center. (2014). The importance of evaluating the impact of continuing nursing education on outcomes: Professional nursing practice and patient care. Retrieved from http://www.nursecredentialing.org/Accreditation/ResourcesServices/Evaluating-the-Impact-CNE-Outcomes.pdf

Andersson, M., Hall-Lord, M. L., Wilde-Larsson, B., & Persenius, M. (2013). Patient photographs—A landmark for the ICU staff: A descriptive study. *Intensive & Critical Care Nursing, 29*(4), 193–201. doi:10.1016/j.iccn.2013.04.002

California Institute of Integral Studies. Retrieved from http://ciis.edu

Carper, B. (1978). Fundamental patterns of knowing in nursing. *Advances in Nursing Science, 1*(1), 13–24. Retrieved from http://samples.jbpub.com/9780763765705/65705_CH03_V1xx.pdf

Health Assessment and Research for Communities. (2017). Coachella Valley Community Health Survey. Retrieved from http://harcdata.org/coachella-valley-community-health-survey

Kulkarni, R. (2016). Top 5 ways value-based pricing impacts healthcare. Retrieved from http://managedhealthcareexecutive.modernmedicine.com/managed-healthcare-executive/news/top-5-ways-value-based-pricing-impacts-healthcare

Nurses On Boards Coalition. (2017). Home page. Retrieved from http://nursesonboardscoalition.org

Richardson, K. (2015). What is the doctor of nursing practice capstone scholarly inquiry project? Retrieved from http://dnpconferenceaudio.s3.amazonaws.com/2013/1Poster2013/Richardson_Poster_DNP2013.pdf

Riner, M. E. (2015). Using implementation science as the core of the doctor of nursing practice inquiry project. *Journal of Professional Nursing, 31*, 200–207. doi:10.1016/j.profnurs.2014.11.002

University of Utah Health Care. (2012). *Cultivating collaboration: 10 new ways to connect ideas and grow the future of nursing.* Retrieved from https://healthcare.utah.edu/nursinginnovation/docs/2012-u-of-u-health-nursing-report.pdf

U.S. Department of Health and Human Services. (2014). About Healthy People. Retrieved from https://www.healthypeople.gov/2020/About-Healthy-People

CHAPTER 5

Setting Up the Project

☐ Chapter Checklist

☑	Select topic—determine your project's focus.
☑	Develop habits that promote completion of the project.
☑	Ensure your computer is up to the task and you are organized.
☑	Set up a record-keeping notebook.
☑	Confirm your plan with the committee chair.
☑	Confirm your plan with the organization's representative.
☑	Start using social media, start low and go slow.
☑	Begin assembling a team to help you produce assignments—the writing center and librarian—and delegate jobs that save you time for class work.
☑	Set up a calendar with due dates.
☑	Identify your support team and talk with them about your needs. Check in with them often to let them know how your plan is proceeding.
☑	Modify this plan as circumstances change.

One of the most exciting decisions to make about the dissemination of your project is the method that you will use to showcase your knowledge about the subject. Each university has its own requirements for internal documentation that you have met the program standards. Most of the time the methods for documenting internal achievement of program standards are papers that summarize the completed project, a review of the relevant literature, a description of methods used to develop ideas, a summary of results, and suggestions for further action. Often a copy of these papers is kept in the department. Increasingly, you can find examples of projects online. These are internal documents and not generally considered a dissemination of information.

This chapter describes a wide range of dissemination strategies and builds on earlier descriptions. These strategies will be used for external methods of dissemination. Using the core document required by the university, you may find an innovative method of dissemination that will benefit the population that needs and wants to know what you have to say. Each method will be discussed in detail in future chapters. The descriptions here will give some ideas for innovative methods of delivery. You'll be better equipped to select an appropriate strategy to discuss with your advisor. Selecting the best strategy is a combination of collaborating with your advisor, committee, and should be based on your expertise on the subject. Choose a method that best suits your audience and gets you outside your comfort zone, just enough to be interesting, but not overwhelming.

☐ Creating a Core (Capstone) Document

To create the best document, you'll want to use the existing university resources to help you. Understanding how the library works and collaborating with reference librarians is an absolute essential to create the best project. Libraries have many online tutorials, guides, and 24/7 access to chats with librarians. Be sure to use them. They will help with referencing and offer suggestions for formatting tools and many other services.

Next to the library, the writing center is your most valuable resource for a great outcome. Use these centers often when you start to write and periodically throughout the project. Take advantage of their writing help. I recommend *not* waiting until you are done with your finished product to seek assistance. Rather, when you have a full draft, submit it to the writing lab. There is nothing more frustrating than spending hours getting a paper just the way you want it, only to find your favorite sentence or a complete section does not fit into the paper when it is being edited. Also use online plagiarism-detection services throughout the writing process. You will not have any problem submitting multiple versions of a paper to these services as long as the settings are appropriate for drafts instead of a final product.

Dissemination is defined as presentation of content to a widespread audience, in a manner most appropriate for the target audience to be able to access, understand, and utilize the information. Matching the method of dissemination with the population that will benefit from your knowledge and insight is one of the most influential project decisions you will make. Projects for older adults will likely be most effective when they include printed material such as brochures or other handouts, TV and radio interviews, websites, and presentations at community groups. A project done to educate teenagers about a health-related issue will be disseminated online via social media or video streaming. Likewise, projects for very young children may involve puppet or other theater shows. The rationale for the method of dissemination should be fully supported in the core document you create for your university.

☐ Marketing Yourself

As you get started on your capstone project, obtain some resources that will help you make a good first impression when you are presenting your information and make it easy for people to stay in contact with you. Using your preferred colors, obtain personal business cards, note cards, and stationery templates (for print or electronic). These resources will help others remember you and impress them with your preplanning public appearances. A headshot is an absolute necessity to use in electronic media, publicity, and presentations. The university photographer may provide digital copies for free. If not, you will be able to obtain headshots from most photographers. Simply ask for digital copies of headshots.

☐ Fundamental Tools and Skills Needed

Any work begins with a personal computer that is current, secure, and can be easily operated without the assistance of someone else. If your computer is over 2 years old, it may be time to consider a new one for *yourself*. The computer does not have to be an expensive one. A simple laptop that can be easily transported (not too heavy) is enough. Later, when you decide on your dissemination strategy, you may need to buy a microphone (the one that comes installed in the computer is not sufficient), headphone, or software. A basic set of requirements for each type of dissemination method will be presented. Even within the basic methods there are many choices available. Pick a strategy that you find satisfying and will be interesting to you and those who will be using the material.

Securing your computer and files is a fundamental essential of contemporary life. Nearly everyone I know has been affected by some type of security breach. Stealing personal information and identity theft is all too common and always a disaster when it happens. More recent, there are has been a significant increase in ransomware attacks on personal and commercial computers. Ransomware attacks come from vicious cyber thieves who lock your computer files up until you pay money to have the computer unlocked. Prevent anyone from accessing your computer who is not authorized to do so. Also, provide for a backup system of getting your files should your computer be lost, broken, stolen, or hacked Three actions will make your computer and files the most secure you can make them.

First, use complex passwords that vary from program to program. Periodically change them. You will not only be doing this for your dissemination project, but throughout life as well. Second, take advantage of online backups, many of which can be found for a reasonable price. It is not enough to have a secondary storage device connected to your computer. In the event of a weather-related disaster, fire, or break-in, you may lose everything, so use a safe and secure online backup for true safe keeping of your files. Third, and equally important, is a system of gaining new knowledge of software and other programs that you will be using. YouTube is wonderful for accessing all types of "how to" videos and they are generally free. Lynda.com is the premium subscription site that provides thousands of "how to" videos on a wide range of topics. Finally, blogs, Facebook pages, and an endless number of websites can also provide you with needed help.

One of my favorite websites with a blog, Twitter feed, and other social media is Free Technology for Teachers (www.freetech4teachers.com). You will find everything you need to create a unique presentation of your information. Start reading about different types of technology to use early on so you have time to find something that is appropriate and you have time to master the program before the final presentation is done. Many types of dissemination that I hope many of you try involve several simple, but varied, skills or equipment. For example, producing a video requires a good microphone so that you can hear what is being recorded, a mobile device for recording the video, and a set of headphones for editing. You'll also need to learn to organize the video through the use of a storyboard, then shoot and edit the video. Perhaps you will want to add some title slides and upload them to a blog you created. All of this can be done in a day, but its best to plan for a lot more time than a day to get the best outcome. Planning will save time and improve the quality of your work.

A final resource you will want to create and maintain is a journal in which you detail what you are doing. Using paper and pencil works fine. Or you can try Evernote (Evernote.com), a great online tool that has a free version that allows you to share lists you have. Use some method of keeping track of what you are doing, what supplies you will need, and problems encountered and successes achieved along the way. A project is a complex activity that takes a long time and involves many skills, far more than you can remember without the assistance of some documentation of the process.

☐ Program Guidelines

Next to having a reliable computer, ready access to program guidelines for completing your project should be consulted regularly. Your school handbook will describe everything you want to know about deadlines, requirements for the paper and presentations, and much more. Take advantage of checklists to ensure you have met all requirements. If there isn't one in the handbook, create your own.

Meet often with your advisor to make sure you are on track. When you work alone, it is easy to get off course. Projects of this size are meant to be discussed, challenged, and evaluated along the way. If you are worried about someone using your ideas, you can set up check-ins with the people you are working with to see whether they will use your information in the future. Creating a Google Alert will help with that.

☐ Transferring Project Content to Various Dissemination Method(s)

Storytelling

The single most important skill for presenting information is knowledge of how to tell a story. Regardless of the format of dissemination, the presentation comes down to a story. Some presentations will be 15 minutes long, which is typical of a professional presentation. Others will unfold over time, online or offline. After understanding how to tell a story, your story of your project, really matters to the quality of life for the people who will most benefit from your work.

Look around for great teachers; chances are they are great storytellers. Every lecture, book, conversation, and other presentation is a story with a clear beginning, middle, and end. One of my favorite storytellers is Malcom Gladwell, who has a new podcast series called *Revisionist History* available on iTunes. Another great presenter is Dr. Oz. He tells several mini health stories in every show. He is also great at using props and getting the audience involved. He is a great resource for learning about storytelling. There are more listed in Table 5.1.

At the end of the program everyone will have a significant document that meets the university requirements for completing the degree. From that core document you will select very specific components to transfer into a medium that will form the basis of the work you disseminate. You also need to create a combination of materials such as a slide show, handout, and video. Think basic and doable when you are planning and creating these tools, often called *artifacts*. The video

TABLE 5.1 **Storytelling Resources**

1	National Storytelling Network	www.storynet.org/resources
2	Tim Sheppard's Storytelling Resources for Storytellers	www.timsheppard.co.uk/story
3	Fevered Muttering	http://feveredmutterings.com/storytelling-resources
4	The Moth	https://themoth.org/education/resources
5	Storytelling Resources	www.tracscotland.org/tracs/resources/storytelling

will not be worthy of an Academy Award but it will be your work and something special. Be realistic in what you can do and in evaluating what you have done. Test out the usability of the material with a pilot group of people who represent the end users early on in your program. Then you can be more assured that what you create is perfect for who needs to use it.

Public-Speaking Skills

Many experts are terrified of standing in front of a group of people and speaking. If you are someone who is anxious or reluctant to get in front of a group of people and present information, then give some thought to working on your public-speaking skills. Check out resources on campus first. There may be continuing-education classes available for graduate students to help with presentation skills. Toastmasters (www.toastmasters.org) is a wonderful group that helps people develop public-speaking skills. There are thousands of Toastmasters groups in the United States. An excellent podcast on public speaking is the Lisa B Marshal series: *The Public Speaker's Podcast,*also available on iTunes. If you don't do anything else, start recording yourself with your mobile device and analyze your presentation skills.

In addition to projecting your voice and speaking at a speed that can be understood, there are other skills such as engaging the audience, managing stage fright, and speaking to the audience instead of the slides.

Technical Multimedia Skills

Each dissemination strategy has two parts. First, a technical side that involves hardware and software to create the resource and second, the knowledge base required to produce the object. Many people get stuck on the technical side and never produce the educational product they want. Don't be a part of that group. Pick simple technology to showcase your work. Don't overshoot. Be humble in your search for an impressive, yet scholarly, way to showcase your topic and technology.

Many of the early uses of technology I incorporated came from a wonderful national organization called *Computer Using Educators* (www.cue.org). They have an annual meeting in Palm Springs, California, around typical spring break times, March or April. The first conference I attended really showed me how to use technology to its fullest. I learned how to use Twitter effectively in my undergraduate nursing classes by incorporating the suggestions of two young kindergarten teachers who demonstrated their use of Twitter in kindergarten. Their use of Twitter was pure genius! They had students work together to accomplish very specific tasks. For example, the children were learning the color orange. Working in pairs, they would collaborate on how to spell orange and then find something in their classroom that was orange. Working together, they composed a tweet and then once the teacher reviewed their work, they were allowed to send it to the group of parents and community members in their town anxiously awaiting each and every tweet from this class. It really was magic.

Producing videos for presentation online is an incredibly important form of presentation. Vines, or 6-second videos, may be the most challenging of all. But it is possible to convey your message in one or more vines, as people are far more willing to watch an ultra-short vine video than a longer "academic" one.

No video should exceed 10 minutes, and should aim for 3 to 5 minutes if possible. To create a video, use standard Hollywood techniques. Look at commercials and see how even a 15-minute commercial can have a powerful effect. Think of how many days it took to prepare a 15-second commercial. Basic video production techniques include:

1. Storyboard the material.
2. Keep the message simple.
3. Ensure the sound and visuals appeal to the selected audience.
4. Upload to where people can find it and market the video to ensure it will be found and viewed.

Websites

Creating a website is a relatively simple process. You will find many free resources with templates to get you up and running in just a few hours. WordPress (www .wordpress.com) is the most widely used free site for both free and subscription blogs. You can also create a Google site among many more options. Use these applications to create a simple website to host your content. You can go much larger and complex with a web page containing multiple pages, but this is rarely necessary. Start small, don't get talked into doing more than the minimum with technology. Doing too much, especially if you plan to hire someone, is almost certain to take some of the enjoyment out of the project.

If your subject is straightforward, meaning you only need one page to describe it, you may want to create a Facebook Page. It is free and Facebook is the largest social media platform in the world. You may not have the page easily searchable from within Facebook, but you can include a "launch" plan as part of your project, which describes how you will let others know where to find your information.

TV and Radio Interviews

Like producing a paper, video, or cooking a great meal, there is a formula to becoming a guest on TV, radio, or Internet shows. To make yourself known to media outlets, you want to establish yourself as an expert in the topic; a blog or using social media profile, such as Twitter, is a great way to be noticed. Sharing content that is of interest to media outlets you would like to appear on is the first step. Commenting on their websites, blogs, or Facebook pages, or writing to producers who provide shows with your topic of interest will help get your name out. You will need to have patience and a plan to become known over time.

Because nurses are consistently the most trusted professionals (Gallup, 2016), your current credentials will get noticed by producers. Providing them with marketable and relevant material is what they need. When you see an opportunity to provide input through suggesting a story or offering to provide an expert opinion, you become a valuable resource. Nurture relationships with show producers you are interested in when you start your project. Then when you are ready, you will already have a relationship established.

Publication: Article

Unit III describes the process of publishing an article in great detail. You will learn about the steps in planning a manuscript, creating it, submitting, and all the steps in between submission and publication. There is a great deal of content on handling the peer-review and secondary editing process. The work of publishing an article does not stop with acceptance.

Interpretive Art

Using interpretive art is an emerging method of disseminating information. Chapter 11 gives more examples and resources to produce artist content. The website Nurse.com (2015) presents three examples of nurses who use art to convey their nursing ideas. Picard (1995) explores dance as a method of communication.

Slides

The most common form of presentation includes presentation slides, created in one of three common ways: PowerPoint (Microsoft), Keynote (Apple), and Google Slides. All work well but may require some adjustments to be displayed on a computer that they were not created on. Slide presentations can also form the basis of a video presentation. Regardless of how the slides will be used, there are many guidelines available to help you create a professional presentation that is appropriate for the ultimate audience. It is key to remember that the resource(s) you are creating for dissemination will use a tiny fraction of what you have collected and synthesized. Narrowing down your hours of work can be painful at times. Especially if you find your favorite part of the project is not sufficiently relevant to be included in the dissemination method. Templates take a short period of time to create, but they can save hours when it is time to create the actual presentation. You can create several designs and test them out for readability well in advance of any formal presentation.

Templates

The first step in creating a noteworthy presentation is to create a template that is uniquely yours and "branded" to you, your project, and institution. Many universities now offer a PowerPoint template to ensure the university logo is used correctly. Check with the graphic designers or marketing group for information on what you can and cannot do with the university logo. Whatever you do, ask about this. You are not only disseminating your work but the work of the university in creating and maintaining the program where you are getting your degree.

The three most important things you need to include in your slide design are:

1. Use a limited amount of type—remember that less is better. Make sure the slides are readable from a long distance and only include the essence of your message.
2. Clip art should be minimized or eliminated. Instead, use photographs that you created or use freely available art from places like:
   a. Pixabay.com
   b. Unslash.com
   c. Morguefile.com
   d. Flickr.com (This site has a number of royalty-free pictures.)
3. Make sure the slides have all the information people will need to have to contact you after they are created. You can use a personal email address and social media accounts; Twitter is a good social media provider for people to use to contact you postgraduation.

☐ Delivery of Presentation

Regardless of the format your presentation takes, plan, practice, and obtain honest and accurate critiques as you develop the presentation. The more work you can do up front to produce a first-class presentation, the better. This level of preparation also increases your confidence during the presentation.

☐ Evaluation of Presentation

Traditional Synchronous Evaluation

Every presentation can benefit from an evaluation of the content, visuals, and skill used to deliver the presentation. This project presentation may be the most significant presentation you have given to date. Throughout your career, you will make many more presentations of significance. If the presentation is given in a professional conference, there will be very specific guidelines for its evaluation. However, none of the conference evaluation strategies preclude you from asking the audience to complete a simple additional evaluation. If it is not practical to have everyone in the audience complete a specific presentation, then select some people before you begin and ask them to complete your form. It is best to have them do the evaluation as soon as the presentation is done.

Other methods of evaluation can include using applications such as polleverywhere.com and similar audience response systems. Other creative evaluation methods can ask audience members to solve a puzzle. Online asynchronous evaluations can be done with audience response systems, using a mobile device and Google Forms. Ask participants to upload a product of their learning such as art, photographs, recordings, and short papers to share with others on a conference website.

☐ Storage and Retrieval of Your Presentation

There are many methods to use to store and easily retrieve your final products. You are likely going to present the information more than one time in more than one way. It is not enough to email the file(s) to yourself. Develop a storage system in the cloud and in your computer. There are many retrieval applications available. You have spent too much time on the project and presentation to lose it. You can use a Facebook page, SlideShare (www.slideshare.net), or a YouTube channel.

☐ Conclusions

It is exciting to be able to share your work in new and creative ways. You've been introduced to several types of delivery methods. Specific instructions will be given in later chapters. Take the time to look at online sites with archived presentations, such as SlideShare, to get an idea of what is possible. There are new methods of delivering information created daily. Not every method available is detailed in this book, but you will find many possibilities to tell people about your incredible work.

REFERENCES

Gallup. (2016). Honesty/ethics in professions. Retrieved from http://www.gallup.com/poll/1654/honesty-ethics-professions.aspx

Nurse.com (2015). Nursing portrait: 3 nurses share their passion. Retrieved from: https://www.nurse.com/blog/2015/05/18/nursing-portrait

Picard, C. (1995). Images of caring in nursing and dance. *Journal of Holistic Nursing, 13*(4), 323–331.

CHAPTER 6

Group Dissemination Projects

☐ Chapter Checklist

☑	Carefully select a trusted group of colleagues/other students to discuss working on a group project.
☑	Establish ground rules and a timeline for project.
☑	Establish group norms, including specifics of each person's responsibilities, copyright, authorship, and how members leaving or attempting to enter the group will be handled; set up a calendar with due dates.
☑	Have a meeting with your advisor to go over the plan and group guidelines.
☑	Finalize contract and schedule regular check-ins.
☑	Develop a shared virtual site, specifically for the purpose of exchanging information.
☑	Create the infrastructure: setting up your own network.
☑	Schedule regular check-ins.
☑	Celebrate successes.
☑	Assume best intentions.
☑	Cautions about group work: employer relations, romantic or family relations, time zones, history of meeting deadlines.
☑	Consider the impact of life events, different shifts, job responsibilities.
☑	Agree to a group project only after extensive discussion and negotiation.

Group projects can be amazing experiences during which a small group of people with a common goal share the successes and challenges of completing a project larger than themselves. A truly collaborative experience is exhilarating and is often transformational. I completed my dissertation with a partner in 2000 (Smith-Stoner & Weber, 2000). Effective collaborations do not just happen; they have to be nurtured and developed over time. There are always highs, lows, and plateaus during the process.

If you have designed a project using a collaborative model in which everyone makes decisions and has equal input into decisions, then you have a true collaboration. Chances are you are at the beginning of an exhilarating journey that you will be proud of and will recall often for the rest of your life. However, if there is a strong person in the group, who "assigns" tasks or asks for volunteers, you do not have the beginning of a great collaboration, it is closer to hierarchy, with someone else at the top who is not you.

☐ Group Projects: Delegate or Collaborate?

There is subtle yet significant difference between delegating assignments in the group and collaborating on assignments in the group (see Table 6.1). Using action–reflection cycles fosters collaboration. If the group utilizes a traditional hierarchical structure with a group leader who makes assignments and checks back with individuals to ensure they've completed their assignment little collaboration will occur. Using a top-down approach to completing the project may save time but does not usually meet program outcomes.

TABLE 6.1 Differences Between Collaboration and Delegation

Collaboration	Delegation
Goals and actions to meet those goals are determined by group discussions, give and take, mutual respect, and being individually accountable for contributions	A single individual establishes a plan and assigns individuals specific projects with the primary focus on project completion
All members of the group help execute the project, checking in regularly, informing, negotiating, and evaluating the work together	Each person completes an individual task
The group works through issues of responsibility and accountability engaged as a group	Individuals take over the functions of other members who are not completing their roles
Authority in the group is shared	One person is the authority who has the final say on the work

☐ Best Practices Group Projects

Producing a capstone project with two or more individuals greatly increases the breadth of your project. When designing the final project, the scope should reflect the number of individuals in the group. The best projects are focused, organized, and deliver according to the stated objectives of the plan. In order to keep the capstone project moving along, members need to be present and accountable, offering information before being asked. Ensure that members are dedicated to the project, can contribute important skills or have access to necessary resources, and that they indicate a desire to do their fair share. In order to make the group project mentally and emotionally satisfying, each person should have a combination of roles that are both familiar and challenging.

Take the time to assess your own communication skills and work with others to develop their skills (Table 6.2). There are different styles of communication online, in person, via a telephone or video conference. Important words like

TABLE 6.2 Activities to Assess and Develop Team or Group Skills

Type of Content	Link
Online teamwork skills—assessments and discussion activities	www.kent.ac.uk/careers/sk/teamwork.htm
Many training and awareness tools	www.trainingforchange.org/tools
Kingdomality—Very fun personality tools	www.cmi-lmi.com/kingdom.html
Best communication skills	www.thebalance.com/communication-skills-list-2063779
Improving communication skills	www.helpguide.org/articles/relationships/effective-communication.htm
Spotting lies	https://smile.amazon.com/Pamela-Meyer/e/B003M1ABY4/ref=sr_ntt_srch_lnk_3?qid=1489965152&sr=1-3
Website	www.cmu.edu/teaching/designteach/teach/instructionalstrategies/groupprojects/tools/index.html
Gloria Totten's Capstone Group project template	http://capstone.unst.pdx.edu/resources/file/sample-group-work-contract

responsibility, on time, complete, and *equality* are often terms mentioned in discussions of group projects. There are a number of fun and interesting tools that will help you assess your own communication skills, assess your potential for group work, and templates that help when forming groups.

☐ Creating a Group

It is critical to carefully consider whom you trust to share the responsibility and successes of the project. Creating a group is not a matter of informally soliciting people who want to "participate" in a project on your selected topic. In the SHARED model, considerable discussion has already been presented on the S in "share"—which also refers to the selection of the topic. Examples of group contracts are found in Table 6.3 and in Exhibit 6.1

TABLE 6.3 **Roles in a Group Project**

	Role	Description
1	Organizer	Communicates with advisor, maintains communication with university regarding requirements, maintains timetable, maintains files and folder structure, ensures publications are supplied to appropriate university representatives, schedules defense of capstone
2	Writer	Creates the outline, format, tables and figures, introduction, conclusions, and reference pages
3	Writer	Writes the background, method/design, discussion, results, limitations
4	Material presenter	Collects material: Journal kept of capstone activity, collects other multimedia and develops new media for presentation
5	Researcher	Investigates online databases in library, creates properly formatted reference list and organized folder for all references, sets up library electronic alerts to be notified of new publications
6	Researcher	Investigates social media, web-based guidelines, regulations; maintains a properly formatted reference list per guidelines for online resources; sets up Google Alerts to automatically be notified of new resources
7	Other	Assigns postproject roles such as marketing, planning, and other jobs related to dissemination

EXHIBIT 6.1 **Typical Components of a Group Project Contract**

- Roles are spelled out.
- Timeline of major and minor milestones is listed.
- Order of credit or responsibility is determined proactively.
- Frequency and method of check-ins are determined.
- Shared passwords for common digital accounts are created.
- Decisions are made regarding how individual group members can use group work in presentations after educational requirements are met.
- Decisions are made regarding how emergencies will be handled by the group when someone is not participating.

When participating in a group project, the "S" in SHARED can also refer to selecting members of the group. Selecting a topic is likely to go from your original idea to a modified version as members negotiate after asking a trusted group of students to discuss working on a group project.

The SHARED model also provides an effective method for determining how a group might work together. Here is a set of questions guided by the model to discuss with others forming your group:

S = Select

- What topics are you interested in?
- What is the population you are interested in?
- What clinical practice area will the project be carried out in?

H = Habits

- What is your work schedule?
- When are you available to work?
- What computer operating system and social media do you use?
- How do you get help with your schoolwork when you need it?

A = Assess

- What resources would you bring to this project?
- What challenges do you foresee with this project?
- How much time do you have available for this project?
- When do you plan to graduate?
- Do you have financial resources, if costs arise, such as traveling to a conference to present the project?
- How supportive is your support system if you need to work on days off or if have expenses related to the project?
- What are your expectations on "claiming credit" for this group work?

R = Record

- During the conversations/negotiations, take note of who is present, what is decided, and what is left to decide.
- Are you able to find notes, files, and other material when asked?
- What backup systems do you use for important information?

E = Enthusiasm

- What is your experience with group projects?
- How are you feeling about the doctoral program?
- Is this a topic/project you can be enthusiastic about?

D = Dissemination

- Remember, if the DNP capstone is not disseminated it was not done.
- Ensuring you leave the time and energy for dissemination, in whatever method you choose is important. Just like charting: If it wasn't charted it wasn't done. If a final project is not shared or disseminated it may as well have not been done.
- A group project is a way of sharing the joy and responsibility of the project.

☐ Establish Ground Rules and Timeline for Project

Be sure you understand each step in the process of ensuring that individual members receive credit for the capstone project. Check with your advisor and the graduate department at your university often.

As a potential group, it is best for everyone to sit down and consider the university deadlines, vacation schedules, work responsibilities, periods when the university is closed, and your chair's availability, along with other significant events. The joint calendar can be created using many online tools, most notably Google Calendar. I suggest discussing these in real time, however it is done. You will learn a lot about each other while you share these activities. Be specific about the habits that each member has regarding completion of the DNP work. Is the person organized and methodical? Or is the advanced degree sandwiched in between many other activities? Talk about the availability of time, a very precious resource for doctoral students, and how much each person has. In addition to how much is available, when is that time available? Finally, in what time zone do members live? Students are in different time zones for online DNP classes and time zones are a huge problem. In summary, time should be described in terms of the total amount available, the days of the week when available, and times of the day available. The online tool Timeanddate.com will help you determine when it is best to schedule a meeting when members live in different time zones.

There are many practical and legal issues to consider upfront. Ownership or authorship of the project is perhaps the most important. There are national and international guidelines on who claims authorship for a publication. The most referenced guidelines are the "Recommendations for the Conduct, Reporting, Editing, and Publication of Scholarly work in Medical Journals" (International Committee of Medical Journal Editors, n.d.). It should be noted that when you speak with your advisor, ask whether that person is considering coauthorship of your paper or other products of your work. Some schools have a policy about coauthorship and faculty advisors, others have optional guidelines, and some have no suggestions on this topic. Be sure to ask before you begin your project about who will be listed as a formal contributor to the project.

One suggestion for handling attribution for group members who contribute significant ideas, suggestions, or other important aspects, but don't start and finish the project, is to mention them in the acknowledgments in printed or other material. You can only mention someone by name if you have their permission to do so, which is another reason to bring this up before you begin. If someone has to drop out of the project, but has made some contributions, move them from author/creator position to someone mentioned in acknowledgments. The order of authors will be discussed later in the book; there is a formula for deciding that.

At the point of matching the personal schedules with the project and university calendars, the group members may see that a match is not possible. There may be too many competing demands from the members. Don't be discouraged. The process of truly looking inward at your own skills, resources, expectations, and needs is very productive. Explore the possibility of rearranging the group members. This discussion should also extend to your advisor. When you meet for the first time and share your plan, ask for information on the frequency, duration, and method of communication (real-time, asynchronous, computer, phone, or instant messaging).

☐ Meeting With Your Advisor as a Group

Prior to finalizing the group contract, it is essential to meet with your advisor and get buy-in and authorization for a group project. Check the program handbook for specifics regarding group projects. If there are no specifications, propose some of your own. In my doctoral program, that is what happened: My coresearcher/ author proposed a plan and it was accepted. Requirements of the program are often tied to accreditation, regulations, and other standards. Some rules cannot be modified. However, group projects are becoming increasingly popular.

Final Group Contract

Once you have obtained the approval of your advisor, proceed with finalizing the group contract and build the infrastructure to make it happen. Before getting on with the work of the project, take a moment to celebrate; you have made it to this point. You are about to embark on a journey that will be exciting, frustrating, enjoyable, stressful, and something you can be proud of. That is a cause to stop, celebrate, and let your loved ones know you have a major project you are undertaking. Be proactive with your family and friends and include them in your progress.

Building the Infrastructure

Regardless of the type of program you are in—traditional, hybrid, or online—you will need an infrastructure or network to communicate, create, edit, store and retrieve, and track activities and progress. There are many tools to do this. Simpler is always better. The Google suite of calendar, documents, sheets and surveys, along with sharing capability is the most cost-effective and universally accepted, but there are many others.

Throughout this book, there are recommendations for technology resources such as shared drives for files (Google Docs, Dropbox, and others) and calendars. Using Evernote or a similar program will assist in tracking not only the progress of the project but the individual contribution of members of the group. Wikis are also another possibility for documenting the workload and achieving outcomes. Wikis can be used to create the group member contract, reports, papers, and presentation material, among many other resources.

Video-conferencing technology will also help overcome time, distance, and numbers of people participating. There are many video-conferencing platforms, such as Skype, JoinMe, Zoom, or Ustream.tv. Conferences between two people can be done using most of those tools and others such as FaceTime on mobile phones. There may be many providers of video conferencing used in your organization, such as Adobe Connect, WebEx, and others. Because you want to own your intellectual property, you want to carefully consider whether you will use employer video conferencing resources or free tools available in Facebook, Instagram, or standalone programs such as Zoom (see Table 6.4).

TABLE 6.4 Tools for Digital Collaboration

	Tool	Comments
1	Google Docs	Allows for real-time and asynchronous collaboration
		Creates a revision history of individual involvement
2	Facebook groups, varying levels of privacy	Can have ongoing communication, check-ins on progress
3	Video conferencing	Google Hangouts—allows for sharing the deskto,p which can be very valuable in collaborating on papers and other parts of the project
		Skype—allows for varying numbers of participants
		Facebook streaming
		All can be recorded and saved for future reference
4	Wikis	Create group documents, contacts, lists of norms
5	Calendars	Google calendar, Microsoft Outlook, among others
6	General technology resources	Sign up for updates from Free Technology 4 Teachers to find and get updates on new technology (www.freetech4teachers.com)

Sharing Documents/Files

Understanding the capabilities of each of the tools you use is also very helpful. For example, Google Docs has a "see revision history" feature that allows anyone who shares a document to track each time someone accesses the document. This feature also tracks the activities of each member so that all others have a complete record of engagement with the file. Understanding and tracking each member's contribution to the development of the project allows users clarity for determining such important things as author order in an ultimate publication. More important, that revision history allows evaluators to individually assess the contribution of each member of the group.

☐ What Can You Expect From a Group Project?

There are many ways to conduct a group project (Reed & Hocking, 2013). Action research (AR) is a method used to change practices. AR (Dick, 2000), in essence, involves a group of people coming together to reflect on a particular issue cyclically, followed by periods of activity based on agreed-upon goals. AR methods are highly effective in producing systematic and transparent change. *A Beginner's Guide to Action Research* (Dick, 2000) is a great starting place for considering AR. AR can be conducted in traditional face-to-face programs, in hybrid programs, or online. The digital tool that supports AR, at the minimum, would be a shared calendar—shared documents with each individual's reflections collected in one location. Another document is the evolving plan that results from periods of reflection. An example of a two-person AR plan is what I did with another faculty member after attending a professional development program. After attending a daylong workshop on methods of engaging students, a colleague and I identified a number of specific activities we wanted to try in our large classrooms of 80 nursing students. Some of the suggestions we encountered were significantly different than our classroom practices at the time.

In order to systematically evaluate the appropriateness of the speaker suggestions, we came together every 2 weeks set goals for implementing one or more of the suggestions and then reflected on the effectiveness of those we had tried in the 2 weeks before the meeting (Smith-Stoner & Molle, 2010).

In addition to a structure for ongoing communication, it is necessary to have guidelines for communication during reflection cycles and for reaching agreement on all matters related to the development of the project. These guidelines for reaching decisions can be informal or formal such as the nominal group technique (Harvey & Holmes, 2012). The key issue in moving forward with a group project is to determine whether decisions will be made based on democratic rule of the majority versus consensus. When all members are placing their names on a group project, consensus is the general standard of agreement. Consult your faculty advisor for any requirements your university has on tracking discussions, agreements, and resolutions of disputes within your group.

Ongoing, quality communication is essential to the group success. Regular check-ins with honest feedback build trust in the group. Holding members accountable to the group norms of behavior and producing portions of the work must be done with professionalism and assertiveness as required. Allowing individual group members to slide on their responsibilities generally leads to failure to complete the group project. It also presents an inaccurate image of the project and members of the group.

☐ Schedule Check-Ins

Once your program is launched and you are developing individual and shared skills, establish check-ins with group members in real time. This is a great method for continuing to develop communication skills while working on the project. You can use a virtual or real talking stick, meaning each member of the group freely shares whatever is on his or her mind. Each person speaks until he or she has said all they would like to say. No interruptions, no judgment, no speaking directly to a person, only the group. The discussion is private and not shared outside the group. A virtual way of doing this is to create a slide, graphic, or photos of group members. Put the photo up so all can see. In both cases, whoever starts, the discussion moves to the left until there is nothing left to say as members of the group speak in turn. Anyone who does not want to speak can simply say "pass" when his or her turn comes. These types of communication–listening activities provide the interpersonal infrastructure that contribute to the success of the project.

The coming together, disagreeing, and reaching resolution on difficult and complicated issues can be where much of the enjoyment and satisfaction of the group project is derived. It is an absolute given that some aspects of every group project will not come together as planned. That is the nature of learning. Through ongoing collaboration, honesty and accountability to the group members grows, both as a single unit and as individuals. This group learning provides a rich and productive foundation for achieving the group goals.

No matter what happens, assume the best of intentions of group members, even those who are not meeting the deadlines. No one ever knows what others are going through. Each person must make an equal contribution, or the entire project is jeopardized. The threats involve both the person who overexerts his or her authority and starts to take over responsibilities and the one who does meet responsibilities. The most common cause of stress in doctoral work is often overcommitting to a project. Be sure to communicate when you find the project is too overwhelming or something changes that threatens the project; be sure to speak with the group first and then your project chair. Keeping everyone informed and on the same page is priceless and a professional way of handling the inevitable conflicts and seeming catastrophes that sometimes occur.

☐ Celebrate Successes

There is life after your doctoral project. Review your group timeline and add in celebrations, however small, for each step that is finished. Assembling your group, agreeing on your topic, obtaining approval for the project, finishing classes, you name it. Keep a photo of who motivates you by your computer. These people can celebrate with you—wherever they are. Make sure you share your successes with loved ones with whom you have shared your frustrations and other intense emotions. Let them know you are alright and you will be done one day. Change is hard.

☐ Conclusions

Group projects are increasingly popular in higher education. The completion of my doctorate with a partner was a very enjoyable and challenging journey. Group projects allow for a deeper exploration of the topic and achievement of greater outcomes. Individual members of the group will need to take responsibility for their individual portions and participate fully in the group actions to bring about a single set of shared outcomes. There are peaks and valleys to the workings of every group, but these can be overcome by planning, respect for one another, and ongoing engagement with the capstone project plan.

REFERENCES

Dick, B. (2000). *A beginner's guide to action research* [Online]. Retrieved from http://www.aral.com.au/resources/guide.html

Harvey, N., & Holmes, C. A. (2012). Nominal group technique: An effective method for obtaining group consensus. *International Journal of Nursing Practice, 18*(2), 188–194. doi:10.1111/j.1440-172X.2012.02017.x

International Committee of Medical Journal Editors. (n.d.). Defining the role of authors and contributors. Retrieved from http://www.icmje.org/recommendations/browse/roles-and-responsibilities/defining-the-role-of-authors-and-contributors.html

Reed, K., & Hocking, C. (2013). Re-visioning practice through action research. *Australian Occupational Therapy Journal, 60*(3), 181–188. doi:10.1111/1440-1630.12033

Smith-Stoner, M., & Molle, M. (2010). Collaborative action research: Implementation of cooperative learning. *Journal of Nursing Education, 49*(6), 312–318. Guidelines for Collaborative DNPs Purdue.

Smith-Stoner, M., & Weber, T. (2000). *Developing theory using emergent inquiry: A study of meaningful online learning for women* (PhD thesis, California Institute of Integral Studies, San Francisco, CA).

CHAPTER 7

Print: Publication in a Professional Journal

☐ **Chapter Checklist**

☑	Select the journal.
☑	Review author guidelines.
☑	Compose the manuscript.
☑	Send query letters.
☑	Submit the manuscript.
☑	Review the manuscript.
☑	Acceptance and rejection: your next steps.

Publishing your first article is a really thrilling experience. It takes time, preparation, and attention to detail. It's a lot of work with a huge payoff in satisfaction. Once you have published all or part of your project, you will have a permanent record of your contribution to nursing science. Detailed steps in the publication process are described in future chapters. This chapter introduces the general steps in the publication process.

The SHARED model can start you thinking about the publication process:

S = Select

What aspect of your project do you want to submit for publication?

To help determine the publication for submission, review the journals you have cited most.

Once you have identified the potential journals, choose a specific type of format in the journal. Each journal has many types of articles.

H = Habits

How can you incorporate into your schedule the time needed to modify your program assignment(s) into the proper format for the journal you have selected?

A = Assess

What assignments have you created already that can be incorporated into the manuscript?

Can you find a mentor to guide you through the process?

How does the time until graduation compare with the publication timeline?

R = Record

Keep track of what documentation is required by your program.

Use the records you have been keeping on your project to track to finish on time.

E = Enthusiasm

Set some milestones to reward yourself along the way.

D = Disseminate

Share your project through any method you choose.

☐ Overview of the Publication Process

The publication process involves preparing a submission (according to the author guidelines), followed by initial review by editorial staff, peer review, acceptance/rejection, and, if accepted, post acceptance edits. It is critical to the success of your future publication that you carefully select the journal and prepare your manuscript using the specifications required for the journal. Careful selection of the journal and preparation of the manuscript are the two essentials of getting published. The process is described in more detail in Unit III. In this chapter, the goal is to have you consider the possibility of a publication and set up your work so that, if you decide to publish later, you will be ready.

☐ Selecting the Journal

To start the process, make a list of the journals you read as you proceed through the DNP program. These are the first journals to consider as potential sources for publication. Be sure to include the publications from professional organizations you belong to and those that are in your specialty. It's impossible to read all the journals you find, but there is a way to keep track of special announcements and new articles in your area of interest. As you locate potential journals you may consider for submission, sign up to receive electronic copies of each issue's table of contents (eTOC).

☐ Habits

Continue to record topics of interest, editorials, and calls for specific topics in your journal. Take note of due dates, even if they will be some time before you will be submitting a manuscript. Begin to set time aside in your day to develop the manuscript. As you complete course work, you can "set aside" specific components of papers done in courses that could lead to a potential article submission.

☐ Author Guidelines

Each journal has a unique set of author guidelines. Reading the guidelines and preparing a manuscript according to them is mandatory. The quickest way to have a manuscript rejected is to ignore the instructions prepared for you. Take a look at the types of columns that appear in the journals. There are specific directions regarding the length of the manuscript, the number of tables and figures, and the type of article. Some less restrictive columns will provide you with an opportunity to publish a quality-improvement project, critique of the profession, or a personal experience. However, each of these types of columns has a word limit that you must comply with.

Once you become familiar with the types of articles you would like to prepare for submission to the publication, start reading those types of articles. This will allow you to get familiar with the style of the journal and what readers are interested in. In the library, you can also check the metrics in the journal online to see the number of downloads for each article, the other articles written by the authors, and the number of times the article was cited by other writers.

Consider finding a mentor to help you understand the process of publishing. Many nursing professional organizations have a formal process for assisting new authors. It is likely that mentor programs are available in each of the organizations you belong to. Mentors are generally volunteers who are interested in helping new writers. Don't hesitate to reach out sooner than later.

☐ Cautions

No capstone document should ever be submitted to a publication for consideration in the same manner it was written for your faculty advisor and university. If you are required or are interested in publishing an article, ask your advisor whether you can work on developing your ideas as part of course assignments. For example, if you are required to write a paper for an ethics course, and this is the topic you are passionate about, you may consider looking at an ethics-related journal and ask for permission to compose your assignment for class consistent with the author guidelines of a specific journal.

You can also edit portions of each of the chapters for your capstone paper. Write them to conform to the author guidelines of the journal that you are considering as a possible source for publication, find an article with the format and style you like in the journal, write to the corresponding author and let her or him know that you admire her or his work. You may be able to find a mentor in that professional. Even if the author is not able to be a mentor to you, you've made someone's day by letting him or her know how his or her work has transformed your view of a topic.

One thing that new writers are surprised about is the fact that nearly all publications are submitted without the expectation of any financial reimbursement. For academics, the expectation is that time spent developing the body of scholarship will lead to increased pay in the form of tenure and promotion at their university.

Become familiar with university services such as online plagiarism detectors, writing centers, graphic design services, and reference librarians to assist you would literature reviews.

Be aware that not all journals use the same formatting guide; make sure to follow the formatting required of the journal selected. Do not ignore this; the submission will be returned without even being read if the formatting guidelines are not followed. You can use an application, such as Zotero (www.zotero.org), to maintain a single list of references for your topic. An application, such as Zotero, will allow you to sort the list and produce reference lists in a variety of formats. Using such a valuable tool will save you many hours of formatting reference lists.

Query Letters

If you're unsure whether the publication you selected to submit your first article to is suitable for your topic, consider writing a query letter to the editor or the editorial contact. A query letter can save you valuable time waiting for a determination of the suitability of your manuscript in a journal. See Figure 7.1 for a sample query letter.

Submission

Once you're ready to submit your manuscript, usually you will need to create an account on the publisher's website. You can do this at any time prior to completing your manuscript. In the process of creating a user account, you may be asked about becoming a peer reviewer for the journal. If and only if you have time, this would be an excellent way of becoming familiar with the peer-review process before you participate in it yourself. Editors are always looking for clinical experts to serve as peer reviewers. Your current expertise may be very valuable to certain publications. Be clear about your credentials, including certifications, specialty areas, and years of experience.

There are specific requirements during the submission process that are outlined in Chapter 17. Suffice to say now that you can count on needing time to comply with a few additional requirements such as copyright transfers and conflict-of-interest statements. Your article will go through an initial screening by an assistant editor and then the editor. If the editor feels the article may be valuable to the readers of the journal, she or he will send the article out for peer review to two to three predetermined experts. Occasionally, if your subject is highly specialized, the editor may ask you for some assistance in finding qualified reviewers.

EXHIBIT 7.1 **Query Letter**

Dear (Editor's name),

I would like to introduce myself to you. I am an advanced practice nurse completing my doctorate. The focus of my project has been on providing patient- and family-centered care to people who are dying on my medical–surgical unit. During the process of obtaining my doctorate, I completed a quality-improvement project that looked at noise levels in the environment of care.

The article is a clinical practice description of a change in care. The theoretical model utilized for this study was Watson's Caring Theory, as that is the theory used by our organization. I would like to submit the article to your journal as its focus is on palliative and end-of-life care. I anticipate the article will be ready for submission in 4 months.

Do you feel this article has a potential place in the Journal of XXXXX?

Thank you for your time and attention to this query.

Sincerely,

your name

Reviews usually take 6 to 8 weeks or longer to consider a manuscript. You may be able to track the progress of your manuscript online at the publisher's website. If you go more than 6 weeks without any communication from the editor or editorial assistant, it is appropriate to call or email either of them for an update on the manuscript. When you receive the reviewer's comments and recommendation regarding publishing, you should expect to be treated respectfully. You will never know the names of the reviewers, which guards your privacy and theirs.

Most reviewers work hard to provide meaningful feedback to authors. If you don't understand the peer-reviewer's comments or you disagree, speak directly with the editor in a professional and calm tone. It may be that peer reviewers are incorrect about some of their recommendations; however, that is the call of the editor.

If at any time during the review process you decide you no longer want to publish in that journal, you can ask to have the article removed. Asking to have the article withdrawn is far better than continuing the peer-review process. Remember that it is never acceptable to submit a manuscript to more than one journal at a time. As mentioned, the review process does take time and some peer reviewers are more punctual than others. Many peer reviewers are academics and their schedules will be heavier during the beginning and ending of academic terms. Likewise, many may not accept peer-review assignments during their vacations.

In addition to the reviewers not knowing who you are, they also do not know who the other reviewers are. It is possible that you will receive conflicting comments about the quality and worthiness for publishing of your manuscript. Editors can assist you in understanding conflicting comments and will be interested in your evaluation of the merits of each reviewer's comments. It will always be your choice to make edits as requested or withdraw the manuscript from consideration.

☐ Enthusiasm

The process of creating, submitting, and having an article evaluated can take time. During the process of submitting your first article you will learn a lot about the process. Sometimes the process leads to publication, sometimes not. The critique you will receive is a valuable form of feedback. Take it as such. Respond professionally to the feedback and ask questions about any specific feedback to the manuscript.

☐ Acceptance

When your article is accepted for publication your work is not done. There will be several activities you must complete in a timely manner such as responding to additional edits as well as adding any new knowledge that occurs between the time of acceptance and publication. It is important to respond quickly to any requests for additional information even if the publication date is several months away. It is advisable to use your personal email as your primary contact when submitting an article for review as you may not be using your institutional or university email when the follow-up requests are being made.

☐ Rejection

In the event your article is rejected, take a deep breath and read the editor's comments. Well over half of articles are rejected due to formatting issues, not content. If you're following the table of contents online and reading the journal, it may be that your topic was similar to an article in process. Another common reason for rejection is the article does not clearly state the new information it adds to the specialty. Nearly every author I know has been rejected because the article does not fit the mission of the publication. Finally, there are times when editors change during the process and the new editor has different feelings about the fit of your manuscript. This happened to me once and it was frustrating to have spent over a year working on an article only to find that the acceptance was withdrawn.

Any rejection should not be a cause to lessen your enthusiasm for the topic or the publication process. Use the feedback received in your rejection to improve your writing. The fix to the article may be as simple as hiring an editor to assist you with grammar and organization. Once you've received a rejection and clarified with the editor that you are not able to resubmit if you make the edits requested by the reviewers, you are free to submit the manuscript to any other journal.

☐ Publication

Once the article is finalized by the editor and publisher, it will usually be available online before the print edition is released. You may receive one or two copies of the print journal. This is less important as more and more journals provide full text access online. Be sure to celebrate this accomplishment. It is a fair amount of work to publish an article. It is a relatively rare occurrence in most nurses' lives and is cause to reflect on all you've learned. If you've already graduated, be sure to send a copy to your school as it is an important example of student work.

☐ Conclusions

It is entirely possible for you to utilize work you've created during your doctoral education to publish. The process for each journal is clear and transparent. The blind-review process is meant to ensure your article receives a fair review. Your unique insight and hard work are something to be shared. By taking time to plan ahead, you can save yourself a great deal of time at the end of the DNP program to prepare a manuscript for submission.

CHAPTER 8

Print: Publication in Lay Magazines, Newsletters, or Other Sources

☐ Chapter Checklist

☑	Select your topic.
☑	Identify the types of lay publications that are relevant.
☑	Understand the process of submitting an article.
☑	Develop your reputation as an expert in the field.
☑	Consider value-added content: social media.

☐ Publishing Your Topic Internally

There are few things more exciting than seeing your byline in a published article in a community publication well known to your family and friends. The sense of personal satisfaction that comes from appearing in a noted magazine, website, or blog is every bit as exciting as being published in a professional journal.

The process of being published in a popular or lay journal is similar to the process of publishing in a professional journal with some significant differences. The similarities are that you must select the appropriate journal that is focused on your content and has readers who would be interested in your topic. The difference is the peer-review process is not structured. The articles are generally shorter and are not full of scientific terms (see Table 8.1).

TABLE 8.1 Standard Process for Publishing in a Professional Journal

	Steps in Developing an Article for Publication	Add Your Comments
1	Select an important topic	
2	Thoroughly collect evidence while refining the topic	
3	Theoretical framework used to guide the topic	
4	Manuscript edited to be concise, interesting, and grammatically correct	
5	Tables summarize and present essential information	
6	Figures are creative, standalone, and memorable	
7	Create a manuscript that flawlessly matches the author guidelines	
8	Gaps, contradictions, and controversies are discussed and solutions are proposed	

☐ Topic Selection

Within your capstone project there is a wide variety of large and smaller topics relevant to your project. Throughout your program, you have probably done course assignments that require you to delve into the issues of your local community. These issues may be health related, political, environmental, or cultural. Articles specific to your community are the most likely to be of interest to lay publications. It is absolutely critical to become familiar with editors, reporters, and other staff at the publications where you feel you may be able to offer some valuable information that would interest or improve the lives of readers. Even as a student going through the program you may find topics you would like to publish in traditional journals. You can use course related assignments as a basis for a publication (Smith-Stoner, 2011).

Lay journals and other publications place a greater emphasis on visuals to accompany articles. If you have photographs, images, or other multimedia, be sure to describe those resources to the editor when you pitch your article idea. I suggest sending a pitch or modified query letter to the editorial contact at the community-based publication before you take the time to compose the entire article. This will save you a great deal of time and frustration if you are not able to find a source for publication. Use all types of sharing tools to let people know about your work (see Table 8.2).

TABLE 8.2 Types of Additional Resources for Manuscripts

Resources	Chapter
Audio files	5, 10
Video	5, 11
Poster/handout	20
Infographic	20
Blog	24
Website	10

Once you have an editor interested in your topic, it is important to stick to the agreed-upon schedule for submitting the manuscripte . Editors will generally save space for an article they have approved. If you're unable to submit the article on time, the editor can have a serious problem filling that space. You may lose your potential to be a recurring contributor to the publication if you're not able to keep your time and space commitments.

You may be delighted to find that several publications offer a small stipend for work that is accepted. It's totally appropriate to ask about reimbursement prior to submitting your article for consideration (Smith-Stoner & Miller, 2010).

☐ References

With all publications, it is important to show evidence to support your conclusions. Lay publications do not have the same standard for comprehensive references, but editors will expect that the content is accurate. Most of the time they will request you only include the most important references with your article. However, you should be prepared to show all of the sources you consulted in the preparation for the publication should any questions arise at a later time.

Social Media

The more you can provide content and sources by sharing additional information via social media, the more desirable your content will be. This is especially true when using visuals and multimedia resources you may have created to support the article. Articles, blog postings, and other media that have images and videos attached to them are shared much more frequently than those without such content.

☐ Conclusions

Choosing to disseminate your project via lay publications may be the most relevant way to provide the stakeholders who were the object of your project with needed information. A lay publication is less structured than a professional publication, but has strict acceptance guidelines. Complying with all the requests, short turnaround times, and other requests on the part of the editor, may make you a valued recurring contributor.

REFERENCES

Smith-Stoner, M. (2011). Developing new writers: Answering the call for student manuscripts. *Dimensions in Critical Care Nursing, 30*(3), 160–163.

Smith-Stoner, M., & Miller, C. (2010). *First responders and the "silver hour."* Retrieved from http://www.emsworld.com/article/10319329/first-responders-and-silver-hour

CHAPTER 9

Digital Media: Websites, eBooks, Podcasts, and Video

☐ Chapter Checklist

☑	Prepare media for the Internet.
☑	Include future plans in deciding about the choice of media.
☑	Invest the time and effort into understanding the web.
☑	Decide among ebooks, blogs, and websites.
☑	Determine the advantage between audio and video media.

☐ The Scope of Digital Media

It has never been easier for a technological novice to produce content for the web. You may be surprised by how straightforward it is to create a blog or channel for presenting your work. Education is about stepping outside your comfort zone. By planning ahead, you can learn a new way of presenting information. The tools needed are generally free and there is a wide range of tutorials available to help you master the basics.

☐ Preparing Your Media for the Internet

Create a blog or website that primarily includes commentary with some images. This can come in many forms. Facebook is the most popular media platform on the Internet. A website like Wordpress can be used to house a variety of material, including text, links, images, and Google sites or many other media platforms.

Something you will have to consider when preparing material for Internet content is the need to appeal to the audience that you most want to consume your material. Generally, that means only the key content is included with links to more detailed information. Whatever site you use (Facebook, Pinterest, or Instagram) make sure it is highly visual suggesting that images are included and are both interesting and support the content.

You will find that you do not need to purchase any hardware as most material you will need can be downloaded from the Internet or created from your mobile device. The file types you can create from your mobile device include photographs, audio, and video files. The quality of what can be done from your mobile device is sufficient for use in a basic website. Have some fun with this part of dissemination. The exact directions on how to produce this content are covered in Chapters 24 and 25.

☐ Consider Career Goals

While you are deciding which of the methods of dissemination you'll choose, consider your long-term career plans. If becoming a consultant or an entrepreneur in something you think you may like to do, consider investing more time in creating a brand through a website. It's not necessary to spend a lot of money or learn computer programming. Keeping things simple is perfectly fine if the design is professional. A website or blog is all about the quality of the content.

☐ Understanding the Internet

A fundamental fact of the Internet is that it is constantly evolving. There is no possibility of mastering the entire Internet. What is more important to understand is that you can select specific tools, create meaningful content, share it, and realize that there will always be a new way to do the very same thing every year or so. It's not necessary to respond to every new application or resource. As an initial step in disseminating your capstone project, focus on content first and design second. There are instructions in this book on how to produce basic content. Thus far, the focus has been providing a comprehensive introduction to the most commonly used tools for content creation from existing information.

☐ Websites

Websites come in many types and formats. A Facebook page is a simple and very effective method of presenting your project. Facebook is the most popular social media tool and is constantly improving the services provided to users. At the other end of the website continuum, you can develop a full website with as many bells and whistles as you want and have time for. I caution you against paying a web designer to do the work. Generally speaking, it is not necessary to go to this extent for dissemination of a capstone project. Programmers may oversell what

TABLE 9.1 Websites

1	Wordpress	http://wordpress.com
2	Google blog/Google+	http://google.com
3	Wix	http://Wix.com
4	Facebook Page	www.facebook.com/pages/create
5	Tumblr	www.facebook.com/pages/create
6	Pinterest	http://pinterest.com

is needed on a website. The more time spent talking with a designer is time away from ensuring the content is created in an easily accessible way. Table 9.1 lists some popular blogging platforms that have free versions.

☐ eBooks

Producing ebooks is far simpler than you may imagine. You can take your capstone project as is and submit it to the Amazon ebook service for anyone to download. It is your choice to choose how you want to present your project, the cover design, length, and price, if you choose to sell it. Amazon has a very well-designed support system for helping you create an ebook through its Kindle Direct Publishing (https://kdp.amazon.com) program. By publishing through Amazon or other ebook outlets, you maintain copyright. The editing required for your capstone project will be simple and more focused on creating an ebook or self-published paper book, rather than changing content to meet a publisher's requirements. It is not difficult, but does require some time to learn. The work needed to prepare your paper for a Kindle ebook can also be outsourced to one of many agencies that specialize in preparing existing documents for ebooks. Table 9.2 lists some

TABLE 9.2 Resources for Creating eBooks

1	Kindle Direct Publishing	https://kdp.amazon.com
2	Kindlepreneur	https://kindlepreneur.com
3	Series by Kristen Eckstein	http://amzn.to/2bf038L
4	SassyZenGirl—Digital Nomad Lifestyle	www.youtube.com/watch?v=k1UddId7Rw8
5	Creative Penn	www.thecreativepenn.com

resources for learning to create ebooks. CAUTION: Do not buy programs, webinars, or publications from the providers of this information. If you are only doing one ebook for your capstone project, you do not need to spend any money. Learning the very basics is all you need to know.

☐ Audio Files

Disseminating your message through audio files has a lot of advantages. The file size is much smaller than for videos, they can be easily edited on a mobile device, and distributed without using excessive bandwidth. If you decide to use audio files to disseminate your information, consider looking into podcasting (Andrejco, 2017; Marrocco, Wallace Kazer, & Neal-Boylan, 2014; McSwiggan & Campbell, 2017). There are many resources available through which to learn the basics of audio file creation, editing, and uploading on the Internet. Once you have five episodes, you may want to consider uploading them to one of the many podcast directories. Table 9.3 lists the applications available to create and edit sound files. You will find information on how to create graphics for title slides in Chapter 11.

Audio files work best when they are created in .wav format. Be sure the program and device you are using makes it possible to easily download sound files, so you can edit the files and upload them to the source consumers will use to download them. Directions for creating sound files are available from LPX (http://bit.ly/2beYyaR).

☐ Videos

You will be able to produce simple videos using your mobile device that will be very effective in supporting your dissemination efforts. It may be beneficial to purchase

TABLE 9.3 Creating Audio Files

1	Audio recorder	https://play.google.com/store/apps/details?id=com.sonymobile.androidapp.audiorecorder
2	Smart voice recorder	https://play.google.com/store/apps/details?id=com.andrwq.recorder
3	Titanium recorder	https://play.google.com/store/apps/details?id=hr.titaniumrecorder.android.free&hl=en
4	Garageband (IOS only)	http://apple.co/2aR1LJA
5	Quick recorder	http://apple.co/2bqodea
6	Podcasting and blogs	http://brandongaille.com

a small accessory microphone for your mobile device. If you plan on recording in an area with a lot of background noise there are editing tools available for resources in Table 9.4 and various resources are available through social media, YouTube, and many websites.

There are a few important basic rules about producing videos. They are:

1. The total length of the video should be around 3 minutes.
2. Everyone in the video should have given their permission to participate.
3. I recommend showing the final product of the video to all the people in it for final approval.
4. Plan your video carefully using a storyboard so that the content is concise and effective.
5. Upload to your Google account and to YouTube.

TABLE 9.4 **Video Resources**

Video Tool Examples and Resources	URLs
Exemplars of videos: TED Talks Thinks Big Series	Ted.com www.youtube.com/watch?v=328wX2x_s5g
Paul Bloom cognitive psychologist	www.youtube.com/watch?v=328wX2x_s5g
Justin YouTube Channel	www.youtube.com/watch?v=g8a4F6mVX64
Animation examples (application creation is no longer available): xtranormal	www.youtube.com/watch?v=k7VH9ykZSB0 &index=52&list=FLDWZIVtydvuM8FODUmT Dmdg
Video Creation	
iPhones/iMovie	http://apple.co/2bqphyE
Windows Movie Maker	www.windows-movie-maker.org
Quick	https://play.google.com/store/apps/ details?id=com.stupeflix.replay&hl=en
Screencapture	
Skitch	https://help.evernote.com/hc/en-us/ articles/214920608
PicPick	http://ngwin.com/picpick
Animation	
GoAnimate	https://goanimate.com
Pivot Animator	http://pivotanimator.net

6. You may want to consider disabling comments.
7. Include images, graphics, and photographs to augment your message. See the comprehensive list of copyright and royalty-free graphic resources in Chapter 22.

More information on how to create videos will be covered in Chapter 24.

☐ Conclusions

There are many exciting ways of producing digital and multimedia content to disseminate your message independently or to support you explaining in real time the importance of your project and its implications to improving the lives of others. Start slow and plan modestly for your initial product development. You can do it. You do far more technical things in your job as an advanced practice nurse than are required to produce the content described in this chapter. Don't be afraid to reach out and get help if needed.

REFERENCES

Andrejco, K. (2017). Social media in nurse anesthesia: A model of a reproducible educational podcast. *AANA Journal, 85*(1), 10–16.

Marrocco, G. F., Wallace Kazer, M., & Neal-Boylan, L. (2014). Transformational learning in graduate nurse education through podcasting. *Nursing Education Perspectives, 35*(1), 49–53. doi:10.5480/10-421.1

McSwiggan, L. C., & Campbell, M. (2017). Can podcasts for assessment guidance and feedback promote self-efficacy among undergraduate nursing students? A qualitative study. *Nurse Education Today, 49*, 115–121.

CHAPTER 10

Multimedia: Give Television and Radio Interviews Like an Expert

☐ Chapter Checklist

☑	On- air media
☑	SHARED model
☑	Interviews
☑	Body language
☑	Terminology
☑	Concluding an interview
☑	Interviewing someone else

Nurses are needed for all types of media interviews. Once you've established your expertise on your topic, you may be contacted by news organizations when a relevant issue comes up related to your topic. More common, you will need to seek out reporters to get your message out. This is especially true if you are working with smaller community organizations that may not have a public relations department to help publicize a community event you are planning or participating in. The information in this chapter is meant only to help you prepare for interviews related to your project. There are other types of interviews relevant to nurses, specifically crisis communication after disasters or other high-profile events. Interviews during those types of situations should follow your agency protocol and employees should avoid reporters unless they know they have the proper authorization to be speaking to staff.

☐ SHARED Model and Interviews

S = Select Topics

Like the multimedia projects introduced in Chapter 10, topics presented via radio or television interviews require the same precision in planning and to ensure brevity. Whether you are pitching an idea to a radio or TV station, you need to focus on media outlets that have an interest in your topic. In this instance, you want to identify your topic, work on your project, and then find the appropriate market for sharing your essential messages. You can find the best media outlet for your message by watching the shows with content most similar to your message. It's not necessary to watch every show. You can search using a hashtag or watch trailers of shows online. Social media, such as Twitter, is used heavily by news outlets and broadcasters. Because nurses are continuously valued as trustworthy professionals, lead with your expertise as a nurse. Then relate what you are offering to an existing initiative or explain how a new topic is valued added and has the potential to increase market share.

H = Habits

Being brief, interesting, while providing important content is a specific skill. Start by developing an "elevator speech" about your project. An elevator speech got its name because an average elevator ride is about 30 seconds. You should be able to discuss your topic in the time it takes to ride the elevator. Elevator speeches take practice. Not only do they need to be informative and interesting, the perfect elevator speech is full of the who, what, where, and why of your project. It will take practice to develop the habit of speaking succinctly with your unique style. The words you use, the metaphors, analogies, and examples must be carefully developed. The presentation takes practice and develops over time.

A = Assess

Matching your message to the broadcast medium you are thinking about requires listening and watching. TED talks are an excellent place to start. Recognize many TED talks last around 10 to 15 minutes. Most on-air presentations take around 7 minutes. You will need to assess your content and isolate the most important points. This is the content only *you* can present.

R = Record

Record yourself, both audio and video, and watch yourself. Do your body movements detract from your message? Is your speech clear and free from any extra filler sounds (Smith, 2016)? Any recording you create should reflect you as a professional. Sounding natural and authentic is important. Here are two of my favorite TED Talks that show the power of personal experience:

Joshua Prague: "In Search of the Man Who Broke My Neck"
Mara Abbott: "The Privilege of a Broken Heart"

TABLE 10.1 Resources for Learning How to Be Interviewed

1	American Nurses Association	http://ana.nursingworld.org/mods/archive/mod230/cernfull.htm
2	Huffington Post	www.huffingtonpost.com/andre-bourque/3-things-to-do-to-prepare_b_6295132.html
3	American College of Emergency Physicians	www.acep.org/Advocacy/Effective-Media-Interview-Techniques
4	*Inc* Magazine	www.inc.com/young-entrepreneur-councilac/5-secrets-to-nailing-your-first-media-interview.html
5	Elsevier	www.elsevier.com/connect/11-tips-for-giving-a-great-interview
6	Become a Social Media Expert	www.youtube.com/watch?v=Kgc23dz2Xj4
7	American Geophysical Society	http://sharingscience.agu.org/share-science-in-the-news
8	StoryCorps	https://storycorps.org
9	The Moth	https://themoth.org/stories
10	The Public Speaker: Quick and Dirty Tips	www.quickanddirtytips.com/public-speaker

E = Enthusiasm

If you listen to the two talks I suggested, you will hear how much passion the speakers have. They are speaking from the heart. They are both experts in their own right. You can follow them on social media to learn more. Your voice, your tone, your body language (even if on the radio) lets the listener know how engaged you are in your own topic. Being sincere, as in the two examples, is the key to your message being not only heard but remembered.

The best person to publicize your topic is you and only you! Start in your community or with newspapers, television, radio, and Internet-based news outlets. You will find several potential sources in Table 10.1. Don't be shy! Many people will benefit from knowing what you know about your topic. Perhaps you want to focus on one or two specific aspects of your topic. Setting the scope of what you talk about is your call. Just take the time to locate the best new outlets that will professionally present the knowledge you gained from your project.

D = Disseminate

Disseminating means a lot of different things now, a video can replace a publication or can augment a publication.

☐ Types of Media Services

There are many types of news agencies and they change ownership and focus fairly regularly. Starting local with your outreach is a good idea. You can ask a local reporter whether he or she knows any other reporter who might like information on your topic. The three types of media traditionally had been television, radio, and print in the form of newspapers and magazines. More and more print media is transitioning to online content only. Other types of digital media include podcasts, social media channels, and live streams that can be done via Google Hangouts, Facebook, Instagram, and other social media integrated into other apps such as Periscope in Twitter.

Interviews

To prepare to be interviewed, think of the audience who will be consuming the interview and the focus of the media outlet. In general, using personal experiences and very descriptive language that is concise and to the point conveys the best message. You can prepare for the interview in advance by making some notes of key points from your project that you want to include in the interview. There should be an elevator speech, repeated at least twice in some way, during the interview.

Feel free to ask the interviewer for assistance in how to handle situations that may come up during the interview such as losing your train of thought or getting off topic. I recommend telling the interviewer the one or two key points that you want to make sure are shared. In general, interviewers are very helpful in bringing the conversation back around to the key points you would like to express if the conversation veers off topic.

If you are asked to do something that you don't know about, it's entirely appropriate to say you don't know but you will get back to the interviewer. Refrain from adding extra words such as him in your answers. Be mindful of body language such as nodding your head, which usually indicates agreement with what's being said even if you don't agree. Make sure your verbal and nonverbal communication agree. Always ask where and when the interview is likely to be aired and follow up with the interviewer after that time.

Present the interviewer with the spelling of your name and contact information on paper or give him or her a business card. Offer to provide additional information should the need arise in the future.

☐ Key Points to Being Interviewed

Timing

You may be asked to participate in an interview at any time. Reporters may be attending an event in which you make a presentation, read something you've written in social media, or be referred by someone involved with your agency. It's unlikely there will be a life-or-death emergency that requires an immediate response to a reporter. Keep in mind that reporters always work on very tight deadlines. If you get a cold call from a reporter, simply ask whether you can call the reporter back in a few minutes so you can collect your thoughts and move to a quieter place for the interview.

Only participate in an interview if you feel comfortable doing so. Ask as many questions as you need to. Be sure you know what is being asked and who will be reading, viewing, or listening to the final story. Get as much information as you can before you start the interview. Always get information on who is interviewing you and ask for this person's business card. Develop relationships with reporters whenever you can. You may want to become the "go to" person for reporters in your local community or those who cover topics in your specialty.

Most of the time you'll be able to research the publications you would like to be interviewed for. Take every opportunity to be interviewed, even for the humblest publication with the lowest circulation. If your topic is important to larger news agencies, they can find you. Many use services to collect stories on specific topics and they will be able to find you through electronic searches. If in doubt about what you can or cannot say related to a project done at an agency, consult the public relations department for tips, protocol, and resources.

The Interview

There are many types of interviews. They can be done in person, via phone, in email, or asynchronously recorded and then played at a later date. As you are being interviewed, keep to the topic you know. As your ideas about your topic develop, create a few concise statements that summarize the project and your results. Always tell people why the project is important. Be enthusiastic about your project. Let your voice, body language, and knowledge of the subject matter convey the significance of what you've done. StoryCorps is a project in which ordinary people interview each other. Starting in 2003, founder Dave Isay started with the idea of regular people interviewing each other in a recording booth in New York City. Since then, thousands of interviews have been done and they are housed in the Library of Congress. Many tools and thousands of interview examples are available on the StoryCorps website (https://storycorps.org). Practice learning to be interviewed and interview others by using the StoryCorps model with your own family and coworkers.

Speak in bullet points. Keep on topic using short sentences that convey the most essential and interesting information. If the reporter gets you off the topic, find a way to "bridge back" to your topic (Stewart, 2001). Always give your name and credentials. No one will know you as an expert unless you tell them. Let the interviewer know whether you have any time constraints and ask whether he or he has any as well. Also ask whether a photographer or videographer is going to accompany the interviewer. A great resource to use to find out what the most important words are to use in an interview, or to find the terms "everyone is talking about," is an online resource that collects information on trends. Buzzsumo (www.buzzsumo.com) is a free service that is easy to use. Simply type the key terms used in your project into their search engine and you will see related

TABLE 10.2 Resources for Finding Interviews

1	Help a Reporter Out (HARO)	www.helpareporter.com
2	Radio and TV interviews	RadioGuestList.com
3	ProNet	www.prnewswire.com/profnet
4	Media Shower	http://mediashower.com/blog
5	Expert Click	www.expertclick.com
6	Be on TV	www.itv.com/beontv
7	Interview & Guest Directory	www.interviewguestsdirectory.com
8	American Geophysical Society: Sharing science suggestions	http://sharingscience.agu.org/ways-to-reach-out

content that people are talking about online. If you discover that one of your terms is relevant, be sure to use it in your interview.

The American College of Emergency Physicians (2016) suggests "identifying" a personal experience to support the messages and add one or two relevant statistics that support the important points in your story. Answers should always be short, similar to testifying in court. If the interviewer wants more, let him or her ask for it instead of volunteering information that may or not be relevant to their story. Even more important: The reporter may have a very small amount of time to present the information you give, so make it easy for the reporter to be accurate and engaging with *his or her* audience.

Reporters of all types are your secondary spokespeople. Think of them as part of your extended team. Make their work as easy as possible. All reporters work on very tight deadlines and have only limited control over what information they have gathered makes it to the final presentation. The more interesting and relevant you can make the topic, the greater the chance the reporter's work will be used. If you get asked about something you don't know about, let the reporter know the question is beyond your expertise. Suggest someone who may know the answer to make their job easier. Reporters know they speak to all types of people, many of whom have never been interviewed. Their questions may be aimed at helping you present your ideas more effectively. It is rare that someone will confront you with questions designed to cast you or your work in a negative light. If your subject is controversial, you should get ready for the possibility that difficult questions may arise. If the subject is not controversial, expect interviews to go well. When asking questions, the reporter may also be simply attempting to focus your response or to elicit more than a simplistic answer.

The only negative experience I have had with my publications is one I knew would be controversial when I was doing it. My pilot study on preferences for end-of-life care dealt with a population—atheists—that is often criticized by believers; also, atheists can be provocative about their views. Richard Dawkins (2006), a prominent political and academic figurein the United Kingdom, cited my study in his book *The God Delusion*. As a result, my email and phone messages were loaded with people criticizing me for doing this research. It was interesting that about half the people contacting me felt I had done the research with an anti-Christian bias and the other half felt I had a decidedly Christian bias. Because I am neither a Christian nor an atheist, I felt that in a way the criticism was a compliment to my lack of bias in the study. The calls and emails soon decreased and the controversy was over.

It is truly rare to be confronted with a hostile reporter as I was when I conducted the pilot study on atheists and end of life. I found most people wanted to voice their feelings and rarely asked me about the research. Many interviewers lectured me and presented a story that really did not require my participation in an interview. This can happen. I was grateful for the exposure of the study no matter what. I am an advocate for all people at the end of their lives. When reporters got way off track, I was prepared to build a verbal "bridge" back to my message (Stewart, 2001).

Body Language

Body language matters when you are being interviewed, even if you are off camera. Use body language effectively. Excellent posture and a clear voice spoken in an energetic tone that is easy to hear are essential. Smile and use eye contact for television interviews. Always lean slightly toward the person talking to you. Relax your muscles with mindfulness exercise like deep breathing before the interview begins.

Terminology

Using common terminology is key to being understood. Never use medical or other specialized terms unless you have to; if you must, offer a definition immediately. Use analogies and metaphors to further clarify specialized language. Provide the reporter with the correct spelling of any specialized words.

Concluding an Interview

Give a call to action at the end of the interview. Ask the audience to visit your website, join your organization, participate in an activity, or otherwise become engaged in the cause. Offering a means of contacting you for more information is essential. You can create a Google Voice account for these occasions when you do not want to use you work or home phone number.

Packaging Yourself

Be well groomed, professional in appearance, and try to be comfortable. The best type of dress for an interview on a clinical topic is in your normal dress. For more formal interviews, wear solid colors, minimal jewelry, and a simple hairstyle. Your makeup should also be simple. When sitting, select a place where you can cross your legs without showing underclothing such as the top of socks or undergarments. If you are interviewed at work, make sure the background is not distracting and supports your message, whatever that is. Don't play with anything on your desk while speaking. Chose a place and time when the environment is quiet. Turn off mobile devices and other alarms, if able, during the interview.

Interviewing Someone Else

You may want or be asked to conduct an interview with an expert or to moderate a panel discussion on your topic. There are many sources of information on how to perform an interview. An excellent resource is a segment done with Katie Couric, a nationally known television news personality ("Katie Couric," 2009). Many of her suggestions are similar to those presented here.

Practice interviewing people you do not know ahead of time. Record the interviews and critique your ability to get information from the person you are interviewing.

☐ Conclusions

If you are thinking of including public media in your dissemination plan, start studying interviewers and interviewees. Talk to public relations staff at your hospital or attend "getting to know" you events hosted by local media outlets. A general criticism by the public is that health care experts are not available for interviews or they speak in such a way that no one can understand them. Take advantage of your expertise and share what you know with others.

REFERENCES

American College of Emergency Physicians. (2016). Effective media interview techniques. Retrieved from https://www.acep.org/Advocacy/Effective-Media-Interview-Techniques

Dawkins, R. (2006). *The god delusion.* New York, NY: Houghton Mifflin.

Katie Couric on how to conduct a good interview. *CBS News.* Retrieved from https://www.youtube.com/watch?v=4eOynrI2eTM

Smith, J. (2016). 13 common mistakes people make when giving a speech. Retrieved from https://www.inc.com/business-insider/worst-public-speaking-mistakes-you-can-make.html

Stewart, M. (2001). RN = Real news: Media relations & you. Retrieved from http://ana.nursingworld.org/mods/archive/mod230/cernfull.htm

CHAPTER 11

Creative Presentations, Art, and Other Performances

☐ Chapter Checklist

☑	SHARED model
☑	Art
☑	Graphic design
☑	Infographics

Being creative in your presentation enhances both the experience of giving the presentation and consuming it as well. There are many different types of artistic expression that can enhance the delivery of your message and increase the chances of your audience remembering the key points presented. The more listeners can be engaged emotionally, mentally, and physically, the greater the recall of the content you present. This chapter offers an introduction to some of the possibilities you may consider as you begin the completion of your capstone project. Specifics regarding resources and "how tos" will be presented in later chapters.

☐ SHARED Model

S = Select Topics

Your capstone may be shared via a series of visual media such as a slide presentation uploaded to SlideShare (www.slideshare.net) or a single comprehensive info graphic or piece of artwork that is drawn, painted, or otherwise produced. Often the visual media complements the text or other media. The selection of media needs to focus on the audience that you are addressing. Images, text, and other attributes of the finished product need to be sensitive to culture, age, and issues relevant to the people who you are trying to reach.

H = Habits

Pilot testing graphics and any visual media is essential to ensuring the final product is effective. Any content uploaded online can benefit from a brief evaluation for users to complete. Many sites have a feedback form after a customer service experience or search for helpful information or other resource. While you will be getting feedback from many people, the most beneficial feedback will come from people who do not know you and are part of the population you are targeting for your content. The habit of obtaining feedback from people who use your content will help you continuously improve your message. Another habit is to develop beta or pilot testing (Schade, 2015) and new media first then launch completed websites or other media.

A = Assess

Along with the habit of constant improvement based on feedback, the project will need an ongoing assessment of compliance with university regulations for your DNP program. You may need to educate your project chair or committee on the benefits of using visual media, with a much condensed version of the content from your capstone. One important issue to include in your inquiry is the storage of any digital products you create. Programs will need to include examples of DNP projects to stakeholders and to accrediting agency representatives. Digital media has an advantage of not deteriorating and can be easily accessed online. However, you will want to ask about the file formats and any other technical standards required for posting to a university website.

R = Record

Maintaining a record of versions of the visual products is the same as keeping a record of other products. There will be several versions developed over the life of your project. Like any other changes made, you will want to maintain a record of feedback received. Online feedback forms are the most effective as you can also use them to produce statistical analysis of feedback. Hard-copy feedback forms can be scanned and uploaded to your digital storage area.

E = Enthusiasm

Trying something new can feel like wearing two left shoes. Adult learners do not like to appear as if they do not know how to do something or what is expected of them in public. The challenge will be to remain enthusiastic during your presentation while receiving negative feedback, especially if the feedback is accurate. Don't take criticism personally if the person giving the feedback does not know you personally. Refer back to my favorite TED talk by Mara Abbott (2016), "The Privilege of a Broken Heart," to see an excellent example of falling short of your own expectations.

Preparation is the key to remaining and gaining enthusiasm for your project. Some of the preparation required is listed later on and in the following chapters.

D = Disseminate

Share your project in social media, traditional publication, or other method.

Using Classic Art to Illustrate a Topic

There is a revolution in accessibility of art of all types. Most of the major museums in the world have digitized their collections and made them freely available for educational purposes. There are many repositories of high-quality images that are available to enhance presentations on almost any subject. Although it's not necessary to purchase stock art or quality paintings, it is advisable to leave micro-donations at sites where you have found meaningful resources to use. It is also helpful to the sponsors of the site for you to leave comments, especially positive ones. This increases the ranking of the website in search engines, which increases the ability of the sponsor to obtain advertisers.

Design Principles

While you are planning the dissemination of your project using some type of art, consider this as part of your overall branding strategy. As you design images, photographs, music, and other aesthetic resources, remain consistent with colors, fonts, and other aspects of the material you use. Over time, individuals will be able to recognize you through consistent design elements repeated in a variety of formats. Everything from your business card, presentation slides, handouts, and other resources should include a consistent image that is unique to you.

It is easy to hire a graphic designer to give you assistance in developing a logo or other visual media. The most common source of designers is Fiverr.com, which used to include charges of $5 for any type of basic project from graphic design to computer programming. I use this service with varying degrees of success. I generally put out requests for quotes or "gigs" to several designers in order to get a sense of what multiple individuals think of my ideas for visual content. Fiverr has grown exponentially due to the low cost and variety of creators who can be hired. However, I have a caution: In my experience, it has become increasingly likely that few if any of the designs I obtain I will actually use. Many of the samples on the creator's site are not equal to the quality of the finished product, they are far less than advertised. Be cautious in outsourcing graphic design, although it is essential when you do not have the skills to create yourself. You want to make sure you have the ownership of the final product, which generally is an additional charge.

Graphic Design: Colors

To begin the process of creating a consistent design, select colors that are appropriate for the topic and interesting to you. The colors you choose should be used

TABLE 11.1 **Infographics Design**

Infographics designs	https://venngage.com/blog/infographic-design
Checklist for infographics creation	www.infographicdesignteam.com/blog/infographic-design-checklist
Templates for infographics	https://piktochart.com/
Graphic design templates	www.stocklayouts.com/Templates/Free-Templates/Free-Sample-Templates.aspx
Creating graphics	http://canva.com

for any media that is created related to your project. Use a color wheel to help you select a combination of colors for your specific designs (www.colormatters.com/color-and-design/basic-color-theory).

There are six basic elements of graphic design that everybody uses: line, color, shape, space, texture, and size/scale. It is not necessary to have a degree in graphic design to produce effective visual media. The resources in Table 11.1 will assist you in creating basic graphics to be used in all types of dissemination presentations. By creating visual media, you can be assured that you have not inadvertently violated anyone's intellectual property rights or copyright. It's also fun to let your creative juices flow and develop images that are as unique as your topic.

Photography

Quality photographs enhance all presentations. There is a comprehensive list of royalty and copyright-free photographs in Appendix 2. Like colors, music, poetry, and other aesthetic elements of the presentation, less is more. Many photographs can take the place of the considerable amount of text. Using them wisely and effectively will add a significant amount to any presentation you do whether it is oral, written, or multimedia.

You can find thousands of appropriate photographs in the resources listed in Chapter 11. I do encourage you to develop basic photography skills and produce some of your own photographs. You can even upload the best of the photographs you take to the online repositories you may be using.

It may be necessary to stage activities in order to get the highest quality photographs to enhance your message. Don't be afraid to use a bit of Hollywood in the creation of your dissemination products.

Infographics

Infographics are an exciting new type of visual media. They are used widely in the scientific community to present large amounts of information in a visually pleasing way. There are many providers of infographic templates that will take a minimum amount of time to master. Creating at least one graphic that summarizes your project is almost a minimum requirement for all important content.

Performances

In Chapters 19–21 the details of how to produce a script are presented. As you get started on your dissemination journey, start looking at videos, musical performances, one-act and one-person shows. Step out of your comfort zone and imagine yourself on a stage delivering a well-crafted sketch that both entertains and informs the audience.

If you have been in theater performances, singing competitions, art shows, or poetry readings, consider this a point in time to bring these talents forward to benefit yourself and others. See Chapter 25 for a more in-depth discussion of how to create a performance. Open yourself to the possibility of doing something out of the box to disseminate your work.

☐ Conclusions

Visual media provide effective, exciting, and fun ways to present your content. By engaging your audience fully in the experience of attending a dissemination event, you benefit yourself and others by creating a space and time that is truly meaningful to all in attendance.

REFERENCES

Abbott, M. (2016). The privilege of a broken heart. Retrieved from https://www.youtube .com/watch?v=E41Sy_Spki8

Schade, A. (2015). Pilot testing: Getting it right (before) the first time. Retrieved from https://www.nngroup.com/articles/pilot-testing

CHAPTER 12

Creating a Support Team to Help You

☐ **Chapter Checklist**

☑	SHARED model
☑	Creating the team
☑	Calendar and time frames
☑	Communication and check-ins
☑	Staying on track
☑	Celebrating success

As a student, you have access to a wide variety of resources at your university. These resources include individuals who will help you collect evidence, edit papers, check for accuracy of citations, and many other resources depending on the university. Several of the larger resources, such as the library and graduate studies office, probably offer regular orientation sessions to educate students not only to the types of services provided but how to access them. Check your university's website for information on these orientation sessions.

☐ **SHARED Model**

S = Select Topics

As you select and refine your topic, your ideas about who you need on your support team will change. The ideal team member is one who is reliable, has expertise in the needed area, is enthusiastic about your project, and plays well with others. Start small and add others only as necessary. It is necessary to ensure anything produced by someone else is done in a format and time frame that can be used by all members of the team. *Interoperability* refers to the ability to use a file across platforms.

H = Habits

The most important habit to develop in a team is to develop a clear plan. That means writing information down, sharing it, and synthesizing information you receive back from others. Team members are happiest when they are contributing to the group goal, and being heard in the process. Establishing a system of regular feedback to team members builds a shared sense of purpose.

A = Assess

Think about the skills you need, and are unable to learn yourself. Prioritize these so that if you are purchasing some services, you have the budget to do so. Other important considerations are the availability of additional team members and choosing alternatives if your first choice is not able to deliver the desired product. A very important consideration is the granting of full ownership to use the finished product you have purchased from a person who provides a contracted service.

R = Record

Because ownership is a fundamental aspect of producing your capstone project, it is important to maintain records about who has contributed to your project and what recognition they will receive. Sometimes others who help will ask for a simple recommendation for future potential customers, some will want an acknowledgment, and others will expect a fee. Other important records include keeping calendars and a timeline, among others.

E = Enthusiasm

Because you are working on your project, it's up to you to keep your support team inspired and on target. Expressing gratitude, appreciation, and regular progress reports help build team cohesion. Maintaining a Facebook page, that can be private, is an excellent way to work with your team online.

D = Disseminate

This means sharing your work in many different ways, including traditional publications, multimedia, microblogs, videos, theater productions, and social media.

☐ Creating the Team

When forming your team, consider individuals and colleagues you respect who can assist you and the entire process of disseminating your project. This means that you organize your time in such a way that when you make requests of each of these individuals, they have the time and resources to provide you with their

TABLE 12.1 Support Team for Dissemination

1	Your committee and chair
2	Reference librarian
3	Graduate studies staff
4	Technical support staff: computers
5	Public relations staff to assist you in using logos and other university-branded material
6	Graphic designers
7	Clerical help—typists, virtual assistants
8	Mentors for your content and activity

best efforts. Because most universities have declining resources and the individuals who work for these resources service students and multiple departments and colleges, they have little to no downtime and appreciate planning ahead, clarity of goals, and instructions.

The typical resource team members will include first and foremost your college's reference librarian. Librarians are now routinely available 24/7 through an integrated network of cooperating libraries. You should be able to get assistance fairly rapidly, regardless of the time of day or night. By keeping a system of tracking references and activities, you can assist librarians when you need their help by letting them know what resources you have versus what resources you need.

The second most significant team member is a representative of the graduate studies office. The graduate studies office provides many services for students, including assistance with obtaining and distributing financial aid, scholarships, competitions, and many other activities on campus. Graduate staffing offices are well aware that most doctoral students work full time plus go to school and have families. So once again, in order for the graduate study staff to be able to help you, it's important to allow time and be clear on what you need. Many graduate studies offices and libraries maintain active social media accounts. You can assist yourself and them by subscribing or following these social media accounts so that you have multiple methods of staying current with what resources are available to you.

Other members of your support team include editors you may hire, graphic designers who could create posters or other media for presentation, and technical advisors who may work on your website or other resources such as streaming media that you may not have the skill to do in the beginning (Table 12.1).

☐ Calendar and Time Frames

The best calendars start at the end and work their way backward. Your calendar should include assignment due dates; committee meetings; school and personal vacations; work schedules and any meaningful personal events, such as marriages, births, and other significant events. Regular communication with the team, starting with getting feedback on the calendar and timeline, will help people understand what you are looking for and if they are the best fit for the team. The calendar should be public; it is important to determine who can update it. Allowing members to change due dates has both positive benefits and negative aspects. This can be addressed by addressing rights given to team members. Some can view, edit, or comment. Allowing users to comment can save you the surprises that may come with allowing editing, but still allow you to get the information you need.

☐ Tracking Activity

Evernote is the gold standard application for tracking all types of individual pieces of information. There is a free version and a version for purchase, as there are with most of the recommendations I've made in this book. GoogleDocs, OneDrive, Noteability, and many others allow users to upload, download, and edit files. They also provide an ongoing record of the people who access files. Original files should be secure and not open to editing by others. It's also important to keep the usernames and passwords of all accounts so you are in control of the files related to your project.

☐ Communication and Check-Ins

As mentioned before, regular check-ins with all involved are essential to the progress of your capstone disseination. Check-ins can be done synchronously or asynchronously, digitally, or in person. Video conferencing featuresm such as Skype, JoinMe, and Zoom, are some of the many tools you can use. Other applications, such as WebEx or GoToMeeting, are also excellent. In addition to check-ins, recordings of meetings serve as an excellent record of your performance.

Check-ins include information on activities as well as financial and organizational issues. It's important to verify everything is being done as anticipated, as you are taking responsibility for the final product that will represent your ideas.

☐ Staying on Track

Regardless of how good your planning is, life happens and things change. When you get off course, and this is a very frequent occurrence, you will want to let others know there is a problem. You may have a private issue or something everyone is familiar with, such as launching a new service at work or preparing for a survey or accreditation visit. There are several possible options when a project gets derailed. Taking some time off from school or a break may be warranted. There is no shame in being human as there is a limit to the amount of stress one can handle.

Modifying a project to a more manageable size, with permission from your advisor, could be an option. If you change your project, you will want to let your team know and be clear about their future participation in the project.

Sometimes staying on track means making changes to the team. Be straightforward and honest about your needs; this will help you and others stay or get back on track. There are an infinite number of things that can go wrong with a capstone project. To move forward means you are present and available. If you can't be present, let people know that you can't. More important, let them know when you think you will be.

☐ Conclusions

A capstone project requires a tremendous amount of work. It represents the best of your scholarship to date. No one can do it alone. It is often necessary to ask for help, whether volunteer or hired. Start out easy creating your team and pick each member not only for his or her technical skill, but for his or her skill with people. Create an infrastructure that allows the team to stay in touch and informed about the progress of your project. Let them know that they are appreciated regularly, so the team that starts the project finishes the project with you.

CHAPTER 13

Alternative Forms for Disseminating Your Project

☐ Chapter Checklist

☑	General information on media for the public
☑	Visuals to accompany articles
☑	Online forums and communities

Using local publications, such as newspapers, newsletters, community Facebook groups, fan pages, and other forums, is an excellent way to distribute information on your project when the consumers of these media sources are the same population that was the focus of your project. A simple way to collect a list of potential sources of distribution would be to take notice of publications in offices, waiting rooms, and businesses that you visit during the completion of your project. You can also ask participants what journals or other items they regularly participate in or read.

☐ General Information on Lay Print Publications

Like professional journals, publications for the general public are financed through advertising. Women's health, fitness, and other journals want articles from professionals, but are likely to want very specific content to match their brand and advertisers (Freelance Writing, n.d). As a result, getting published is highly competitive and it is sometimes challenging to be able to publish material from your project in one of these publications, either in print or online. However, if your subject matter and presentation style are consistent with the content desired by the consumers who read these publications, you will have a significantly improved chance of publishing some aspect of your project in any of the relevant consumer-oriented publications, nationally or internationally.

Although publication in professional journals is highly structured, a lay journal has many more restrictions and requirements for formatting, length, and tone. Publications meant for consumption by the public must be generally positive, free of any jargon, and inspire readers by a call to action to change their lives in some way. Many types of articles can be written, but there is a general preference for personal stories of barriers overcome and challenges met; these types of articles are always in high demand.

☐ Visual Images

Another difference between professional and consumer-oriented publications is the latter emphasize the use of color images to support the story. Although it is rare that a professional publication is printed in full color, with exceptions such as the *American Journal of Nursing* and *Home Healthcare Nurse*, today most professional journals appear in black and white except for cover. Lay journals, forums, and social media aimed at the public require appropriate images to be included with many articles. Editors also have access to large stocks of photographs and may find one to include independent of the author's choice.

Assessing Where to Target Your Final Project

As you continue to define and refine your dissemination plan, consider submitting an article or pitching a story idea to the editor of the journal that is of interest to the population in your project. Consider national, regional, and local publications with print and online editions as potential targets for a portion of your dissemination plan. As with all public use of your agency and stakeholder organizations included by name in your project, you must obtain permission to use their names before pitching the story idea or submitting an article for consideration. Sometimes obtaining approval for the use of the name in a widely circulated publication will require engaging in an extended process of obtaining approval. When planning your timeline, make any necessary considerations about delays that may arise from these processes.

Online Forums

During the process of completing your project, you may have encountered a number of online forums that are relevant to your audience. Before posting any requests for participation, surveys, or reports on the results of surveys, contact the webmaster or moderator of the forum to ask permission and obtain the forum guidelines for posting.

When adding material to online forums, be sure to specify relevant dates and contact information for yourself and others involved in the project. Make it easy for forum users to find you and ask questions. Specify how you can be contacted offline should the need arise. It is very helpful to start a second account in social media that is separate from work-related or personal accounts so that your personal information is protected and it is easier to track engagement with others who are following you based on your project.

☐ Conclusions

As you are creating your capstone dissemination plan, consider all possibilities for locations to publicize the results of your work. Many dissemination plans will include both professional and public distribution of information. Each type of publication and online resource has its own unique requirements, audience interest, and allocations. As always, contact the editor, webmaster, or forum moderator before you post or submit any information.

REFERENCE

Freelance Writing. (n.d.). How to publish in women's magazines. Retrieved from https://www.freelancewriting.com/magazine-writing/how-to-write-for-womens-magazines

CHAPTER 14

Internal Publications: Handbooks, Policy and Procedure Manuals, Patient Education Material

☐ Chapter Checklist

☑	Identify all the possible types of internal publications.
☑	Identify the audience for each type of internal publication.
☑	Determine who the "gatekeepers" are for developing any new material or updating existing material.
☑	Set up a timeline for completing your program and meeting internal regulations for developing internal publications or media.
☑	Determine ownership of the final document and possibility of a byline with your name.
☑	Identify the best presentation method for the capstone project and its audience.

☐ Identify the Types of Internal Documents Needed

There is a wide range of internal documents that are used by employees, visitors, patients, community members, and others that can be part of the evidence of completing your program objectives. Review your program handbook and speak with your advisor about innovative possibilities for internal dissemination strategies. Redesigning a skills day or preparing a budget that includes innovative technologies or staffing models for new levels of practice or new services can be a perfect model for demonstrating doctoral-level understanding of patient care.

But there are some cautions to consider. First, many internal documents are corporate property and cannot be shown to a faculty member who is not affiliated with your agency. It may be fine for you to work on the high-level project, but you may not be authorized to share the specifics of what you did. Similar to HIPAA (Health Insurance Portability and Accountability Act of 1996) laws, there are expectations of corporate privacy as well.

Another aspect of ownership that will be discussed several times in the book is how you present yourself when you are completing the activities. Separate your student self from your employee self. Many would suggest you not complete your work at your agency because of complex ownership issues and problems with HIPAA, which I do not agree with as a blanket statement. Many agencies, especially rural ones, rely heavily on existing staff to assist them in moving forward with their quality and other initiatives. Many innovations can only be made by staff who are advancing their careers through obtaining new degrees. Be open with your leadership team and express your concerns. Ask for a written document explaining what can and cannot be done with data you collect about nonpatient topics. Be frank about what is expected of you by your university. Invite your advisor to meet with the leadership of your facility in order to answer questions you may not know the answer to; there are many nuances to university and corporate policies.

Throughout the entire degree process, keep everyone informed of your progress, especially if you hit a snag. Keep documents that belong to the institution there; just like patient records, never take them home for review. Breaches of confidentiality of corporate budgets, future expansion plans, staffing mixes, and other information could have a profound effect on the ability of any organization to meet its mission and objectives. A list of common internal documents that could be used for dissemination projects is found in Table 14.1.

TABLE 14.1 Internal Documents for Dissemination

	Document
1	Policy and procedure—patient care
2	Customer service instructions
3	Patient education
4	Nursing/student education/orientation information
5	Visitor education: etiquette, visiting hours
6	Surveys for satisfaction
7	Volunteer education
8	Children's education
9	Community support-group information

☐ Identify the Audience for Each Type of Internal Publication

Each type of internal document will have a different audience. The people who will be using the document are the audience. Along the way there may be other reviewers or gatekeepers who are involved; they will be discussed later. If the internal publication is going to be used with new employees during orientation, with volunteers, or community members, the document will need to look different for each. Include a full description of the intended audience in your proposal. Likewise, the format may look very different for your assignments versus your final capstone project. Expect that your project will have many versions. From the initial draft to the final product, you will be rewriting the project plan and reporting on what happened. There are many sources to consult to help you design policies and procedure to include in your internal publications (Table 14.2). When you are disseminating your project in the form of a policy, there will be additional revisions.

☐ Best Practices: Pilot Projects Before the Policy

It may take much more than simply rewriting a policy to meet your capstone requirements. It is entirely possible your program will require pilot testing or other methods of ensuring a policy is effective, safe, and evidence based. Before a policy can be implemented, a pilot project generally tests the policy. The pilot testing of a new policy on the day, night, weekend, and holiday shift is an ideal

TABLE 14.2 **Sources of Current Content for Policies and Procedures**

	Source	Location
1	The Joint Commission	www.jointcommission.org/ealerts
2	Institute of Medicine	www.nationalacademies.org/hmd Click on "email updates," to join many of their social media resources
3	American Nurses Association	www.nursingworld.org Join social media resources; sign up for email updates
4	Nurses Wound and Ostomy Care	www.wocn.org
5	Oncology Nurses Association	Offers online databases, creates properly formatted reference list and organized folder structures for all references, you can set up library electronic alerts to be notified of new publications: http://ons.org
6	Patient Safety & Quality Healthcare	www.psqh.com

doctoral-level project. The hospital runs very differently when the usual staff is not at work (Heslip, 2017). The supplies and personnel available to obtain and work with sophisticated equipment, to support the patient and family, and even maintain the environment of care and equipment can vary widely.

Policies and Procedures

There is a large global body of research on the impact of policies and procedures on nursing and patient care (Boise State University, n.d.). Most recently, use of mobile phones while at work in a hospital has been the focus of attention. In a recent study by Cho and Lee (2016), 312 nursing students were asked about their cell phone use and their observations of cell phone use by nursing staff. Nearly half of the students reported using their cell phones while at the clinic and reported having observed over 80% of nurses doing the same. This is during a time when phone use is restricted.

Many cell phone policies are available on the Internet. A major breach of patient privacy occurred recently when staff used cell phones to take photos of a dead patient's genitals (Wenner, 2017). In addition to avoid violating patient confidentiality, cell phone etiquette requires staff to keep phones silent or in vibrating mode. As a capstone project idea, understanding how to best use rapidly evolving mobile technology would be an excellent project. Phones are no longer just phones. They are cameras, video recorders, audio recorders, note pads, and provide many more services. Take a look at all the policies in your institution to see whether they cover the wide range of all the possibilities that need to be covered in the policies and procedures manuals.

Practice Alerts

Practice alerts provide an excellent wat to stay current on policies and procedures. The American Association of Critical-Care Nurses, along with most national nursing organizations, allow nonmembers to sign up for email updates for their practice alerts, so anyone with an interest can be notified of changes in practice.

Another area of research on the impact of policies and procedures concerns death and dying. One research study I coauthored was on the impact of postmortem policies (Smith-Stoner & Hand, 2012). Family presence during cardiopulmonary resuscitation (CPR) is a complicated policy to develop, maintain and enforce, but very necessary (Guzzetta, 2016). Many states are in the process of approving medical aid-in-dying laws, which used to be called *physician-assisted suicide*. These policies and proce-dures will be reevaluated over the next few years. There are many ways to approach implementing a policy or educating the staff and community should your agency reject a person's legal right to end his or her life when the person has a terminal condition.

Patient Education Material

Patient education material is one of the most common types of internal dissemination projects needed. There are many research studies dedicated just to testing the efficacy of brochures with different populations (Ilic et al., 2015).

TABLE 14.3 Sources of Copyright-Free Material for Educational Purposes

	What They Have	URL
1	Photographs	Morguefile.com
2	Photographs, illustrations, videos	Pixabay.com; careful, Shutterstock owns this and intersperses images requiring fees with the free ones
3	Photographs	Flikr.com; search for Creative Commons licenses that allow you to reuse photographs
4	All types of free material, photographs, art, books, etc.	www.openculture.com Everything you could ever want

Educational material can take many forms. For example, children may like flash cards rather than booklets or other printed material (Paulovich, 2015). Flash cards will rely more on drawings than on text. If you cannot draw yourself, you will find many sources of copyright-free material in Table 14.3.

☐ Determine Who the "Gatekeepers" Are

Policy and procedure manuals, educational material, website content, and instructions of any kind are legal documents that often require review by a lawyer or some type of risk manager, which can add time to the completion of your project. Find out who the gatekeepers of your project are and stay in tune with any changes to the process. Typically, policies are reviewed annually.

There are other gatekeepers involved when using material, such as logos, and developing material that will be seen by others. Every organization has a "style guide" that describes the way a logo will be displayed, the type of font that can be used when referring to the company, and many other details about the organization. Consider these details when referring to the organization in your work. For example, here is a link to The Joint Commission's style guide (www.jcrinc .com/assets/1/7/JCR_Style_Manual_CH9.pdf; Table 14.4).

Timeline for Completing Your Program

Keep the timeline of your projected completion date accurate at all times. Meetings are scheduled, canceled, and rescheduled. One meeting may depend on another to happen. Let your advisor know if a critical meeting or event does not happen, so a work-around can be planned. There are always ways to deal with the unexpected when people are notified early.

TABLE 14.4 **Guides to Writing Policy**

University of Colorado	www.cu.edu/sites/default/files/APSwritingguide.pdf
WikiHow: How to write policies and procedures for your business	www.wikihow.com/Write-Policies-and-Procedures-for-Your-Business
Policies and Procedures for Healthcare Organizations: A Risk Management Perspective	www.psqh.com/analysis/policies-and-procedures-for-healthcare-organizations-a-risk-management-perspective
Patient-specific education resources	www.healthit.gov/providers-professionals/achieve-meaningful-use/menu-measures/patient-education-resources
Easy-to-read staff educational resources	https://medicine.osu.edu/orgs/ahec/Documents/Toolkit%20edit.pdf

Some of the readers most interested in the results of your project may be your fellow employees and colleagues. Although an organizational newsletter or blog may reach a number of people in your organization, nothing has an impact like changes to the handbook, policies and procedures, or educational material used by nurses.

The development of an easy-to-understand, evidence-based, comprehensive policy and procedure about an important topic could be a true gift to your organization. Likewise, a well-developed employee professional development course, handout, or other information, such as an infographic, is something that can be consumed by larger numbers of people on a daily basis. Such publications are golden resources that will assist people who share the same goals of quality patient care delivered from an employer of choice in your community. For hospitals that are Magnet facilities or in the process of Magnet accreditation, participation in committees that influence patient care is highly valued. Not only may these activities be beneficial, they may have a substantial positive impact on your earnings.

☐ Determine Ownership

When you are developing something new for your organization to use, discuss who owns the material, especially if the educational material you develop will be part of a class that will eventually a charge for admittance. It is a well-known standard that if you are creating material during your work hours when you are being paid, your employer owns the rights to the products of your work. The ownership is less clear when you are working as a student. You will want to check your student handbook for the rights the school and your advisor have to any ownership, especially coauthorship in publications and presentations.

To keep the lines of ownership clear with your employer, when you are there as a student, wear your student name tag and school uniform, if there is one, introduce yourself to all as a student, and don't work on school projects when you are being paid. Remember to keep your journal of project activities up to date at all times.

☐ Identifying the Best Presentation of Project Outcomes

Take an inventory of the publications and electronic and print resources that you use on a daily or regular basis. Check to see which ones cover the same types of content that is part of your capstone project. Make a list of those publications that complement the work you are doing. Clarify the person or committees in charge of revising these documents. If you are unable to find a document or resource that covers the focus of your capstone project, find out which people or committees are involved in the creation of new resources for organizational or educational purposes for your agency.

☐ Timelines

Timelines can be too long to meet the program requirements for establishing completion of the objectives for a policy and procedure to be used as a terminal example of your work. If a policy and procedure committee meets once or twice a year the deadline may exceed the academic deadlines of your project. Check with your faculty advisor about the most appropriate example of work that will meet the university requirements. Consider timelines for your university and agency before committing to a policy change project.

Formats

Once you have identified the type of internal publication relevant to your project, you will need to speak with the individual responsible for maintaining currency of those documents. Discuss the possibility of focusing your dissemination plan on your work related to improving the existing document or creating a new one. There is a caution here because policies and procedures especially can take long periods of time to be approved. There is generally a multi-layered process to approve policies and procedures that includes internal stakeholders and external experts such as lawyers and public relations individuals.

The formats of specialized types of publications are highly structured. There is no possibility of varying from the established design. This may or may not be an issue with the program requirements.

☐ Publicizing the Resources

You may be required to include a description of how you will go about educating employees, patients and families, or other stakeholders about the new resource you have created. There are many resources within this book to assist you with that. A word to the wise: When you are conducting an internal communication program to educate staff or others, it is best to consider that they have no knowledge or experience with the topic. Treating colleagues and other staff members with the same care and respect that you give members of the public greatly enhances the possibility of the behaviors or other recommendations covered in the document you created being adopted.

☐ Conclusions

Sharing your hard work and interesting insights is the key to moving nursing science and practice innovations forward. Policies and procedures manuals may not be the kind of document that you can download from a library, but many people are likely to rely on them. A well-written policy and procedure is worth its weight in gold and will surely make you a hero where you work.

REFERENCES

Boise State University. (n.d.). *Policy and procedures writing guide.* Retrieved from https://policy.boisestate.edu/policy-writing-guide

Cho, S., & Lee, E. (2016). Distraction by smartphone use during clinical practice and opinions about smartphone restriction policies: A cross-sectional descriptive study of nursing students. *Nurse Education Today, 40*, 128–133. doi:10.1016/j.nedt.2016.02.021

Guzzetta, C. (2016). Family presence during resuscitation and invasive procedures. *Critical Care Nurse, 36*(1), e11–e14. doi:10.4037/ccn2016980

Heslip, N. (n.d.). DOs and DON'Ts of policy writing. Retrieved from http://www.hcca-info.org/Portals/0/PDFs/Resources/library/DOs%20and%20DONTs%20of%20Policy%20Writing.pdf

How do we implement best practices in our organization? (2014). Rockville, MD: Agency for Healthcare Research and Quality. Retrieved from http://www.ahrq.gov/professionals/systems/hospital/pressureulcertoolkit/putool4a.html

Ilic, D., Jammal, W., Chiarelli, P., Gardiner, R. A., Hughes, S., Stefanovic, D., & Chambers, S. K. (2015). Assessing the effectiveness of decision aids for decision making in prostate cancer testing: A systematic review. *Psycho-Oncology, 24*(10), 1303–1315. doi:10.1002/pon.3815

Paulovich, B. (2015). 'The rehab journey': Developing a flash card resource to educate paediatric rehabilitation patients about aspects of their recovery—A designer's perspective. *Journal of the Australasian Rehabilitation Nurses' Association, 18*(3), 10–17.

Smith-Stoner, M., & Hand, M. W. (2012). Expanding the concept of patient care: Analysis of postmortem policies in California hospitals. *MEDSURG Nursing, 21*(6), 360–366.

Wenner, D. (2017, September 15). UPMC hospital cited for allowing cellphone photos, video of Pa. patient's genitals. Retrieved from http://www.pennlive.com/news/2017/09/upmc_hospital_cited_for_allowi.html

CHAPTER 15

Dissemination Through Professional Print Publications

☐ Chapter Checklist

✓	SHARED model
✓	Initial steps to getting published
✓	Commitment to publication in a professional journal
✓	Clarifying program requirements
✓	Your honor *and* integrity in the publication process
✓	Your first conversation with an editor
✓	Preparing for submission
✓	Postacceptance activity
✓	Postrejection activity
✓	Celebrating success
✓	Building a career of scholarship

You can get all or part of your DNP published.

Just like most areas of nursing, for example, preparing a patient for surgery or giving a medication, there is a specific process to follow in order to be compliant with legal and professional guidelines and for the treatment to be successful. The same is true of publishing. The right topic, submitted in the correct form, at the right time, with enthusiasm for the journal and manuscript are the basic requirements of getting published. This chapter goes over the process of successfully getting your work published for the first time. The process does not require magic or graduation from a certain type of school. The peer-review process is blinded to any individual attributes of an author. The process does require compliance with author guidelines and attention to detail.

☐ Why Should You Publish?

You've done great work and the nursing profession is waiting to hear about your success or failure. It is just too much work to get a doctorate not to share what you have done. In some cases, you may share more about the journey of creating the project, writing a "lessons learned" manuscript rather than writing about the actual project. Another type of article might describe how your project transformed your way of thinking about nursing, evidence-based practice, or another transformation that occurred. This chapter is focused on publishing your content in an existing journal. Publishing an ebook or other self-publishing is covered in Chapter 9.

☐ Your Program Requires a Submission—Now What?

For some time, nurses advancing their education have been either strongly encouraged or required to submit their final paper to a journal, any journal, for publication. This trend is changing, however, due to mounting evidence that many DNP students are simply submitting final projects without regard to anything other than obtaining an email proving the manuscript was submitted.

Attending a conference where this issue was passionately discussed among the leading editors of nursing journals was a transformational experience for me and the genesis of this book (Kennedy, Newland, & Owens, 2016). Imagine you are an advanced practice nurse working in a maternal–child unit and overnight, without your knowledge, the administration of your hospital decides that your unit staff will now be responsible for doing all your usual work and educating entire groups of nursing students in the basics of maternal–infant care. There are no longer limits on how many students your unit can take, and when the first group students arrive, only a few are serious about this clinical experience. Many tell you they have to attend but they have no interest in working in the area. This is the situation some editors have found themselves in.

Virtually overnight many DNP programs were created and many had a requirement that students would submit a manuscript for publication as part of demonstrating competence before graduating. Although some editors are also academics, most are clinicians. When the flood of capstone assignments arrived in their journal inboxes "as is" many were unaware and unprepared to provide basic instruction on the mechanics of getting published. Many of the editors with whom I have discussed this situation want to publish DNP manuscripts. They sometime find one that fits the journal and are able to work with the rare author who is responsive to their questions. However, many submissions lack the one requirement of many journals: data. The second requirement is rapid response to staff or editor communication. No matter how unlikely a prospect of acceptance to a journal is for you, I can assure you it is possible and likely if you follow the steps detailed in this chapter.

☐ SHARED Model

S = Select Topics and the Journal

There are large and small aspects of the work you completed throughout your DNP program that are publishable. If you have completed a research study, quality-improvement project, or review of the literature, you will find a home at a journal that specializes in that content. The best place to start is to examine the list of journals you most often used during your program. The best list of nursing journals to consider and avoid is kept by Nurse Author and Editor (http:// naepub .com). This website has a wealth of information for new and experienced writers.

 The best journal to consider submitting the manuscript adapted from your project to is one you read. Journals come in all types and have various needs for submissions. A typical journal has a commentary section in which authors can analyze a current situation in specialty, quality-improvement, and other projects, along with space dedicated to research of all types (Table 15.1).

Timing is everything in publication. Journals have varying frequencies of publication ; not all are monthly. Some published every other month, quarterly, or even annually. Others publish additional supplements on special topics; the only way you will know about the details of whether a journal is the right fit for you is to follow this three-step process: First become familiar with the last 2 years of journal topics, second, evaluate the author guidelines for the journal interest and requirements, third, contact the editor through a query letter.

H = Habits

Being brief, interesting, and provide important content is a specific skill. Start by developing an "elevator speech" about your project. The elevator speech got its name because an average elevator ride is about 30 seconds, so an elevator speech should take no longer than 30 seconds to deliver. Elevator speeches take practice. Not only do they need to be informative and interesting, the perfect elevator speech is full of the who, what, where, and why of your project. It will take practice to develop the habit of speaking succinctly with your unique style.

The words you use, the metaphors, analogies, and examples must be carefully developed. The presentation takes practice and develops over time.

Another habit you will need to develop or enhance is the skill of writing. To hone that skill, one must write habitually. The tools of writing are covered later in the chapter. You can develop your own habit of writing or you can use established methods such as the Pomodoro Technique (https://en.wikipedia.org/wiki/Pomodoro_Technique). The Pomodoro technique is a six step process to write in 25- to 30-minute intervals. Writing sessions continue in short intervals until the timer goes off or the task is completed. It is a considered a highly effective way of completing written work.

A = Assessing the Worthiness for Publication of Your Capstone Paper

There is no capstone paper that can be published "as is." To put in another way: Do not submit any paper completed for a course assignment to any journal. The only exception would be if the paper was written for a journal according to the author guidelines. The reason for this is that educational programs have accreditation requirements and journals have publisher/audience requirements. These different requirements are independent of one another. What is relevant and "shareable" between the two is the content. The paper written as a student will need to be revised for submission. The most important revision is to edit the paper to be read by an audience of professionals instead of the faculty. Faculty are evaluating the paper to ensure program standards are met.

Editors are looking for manuscripts that get the attention of readers; a document that indicates you have mastered program requirements is usually not relevant to professional publications. You will find information on special issues through looking at calls for specific topics (www.nln.org/newsroom/newsletters-and-jour-nal/nursing-education-perspectives-journal/call-for-special-issue-manusripts).

TABLE 15.1 Selecting the Journal and Type of Article

1	Do a search in the library for publication titles. Look beyond nursing to other types of publications that share an interest in your topic.
2	Look for journals of professional associations that may only appear online and not indexed in the Cumulative Index of Nursing and Allied Health Literature.
3	In-depth case studies of complex patients, families, or other organizational concerns are a type of article that is highly valued by practice-focused journals is. Consider extracting an interesting case or example for a journal article.
4	Consider submitting a detailed, focused description of a best practice to a nursing education journal for nursing students to learn.
5	Reformat the paper for submission to a journal so that it is focused on a specific aspect of your topic, such as the theoretical framework.
6	Do not submit to a predatory journal (see Beall's List http://beallslist .weebly.com).

Typically, other revisions needed to student papers include a serious reduction in the number of pages. Less is more in publishing, especially when submitting a nonresearch article.

Reformatting the entire manuscript to fit the style of the journal is one of the first things to do. By reading issues of the journal, you may be identify an article that has a style similar to your own. Examine the article and how it is put together. Write to the corresponding author and let her or him know how much you appreciate her or his writing style. I have made many professional acquaintances by doing this.

When you find an article style you like, speak with the original author to discuss their approach to writing. You may find a new mentor. If you end up incorporating the style into your own paper, let the corresponding author know and offer to mention the author in the acknowledgments of your paper. Many students are reluctant to contact corresponding authors about anything to do with their article. As an accomplished writer, I can't think of anything more exciting than getting an unsolicited email from someone with a comment on my work irrespective of whether it is positive or negative. Anyone who takes time to write to me about my work is someone I want to respond to.

There is one common challenge students face when taking the first step in reformatting a paper written for publication: cutting the paper down to a manageable size. You may benefit from hiring an editor to help with this process. It can be very overwhelming to cut out favorite portions of your paper because they don't fit the journal where the article will be submitted. I have experienced this myself. When I start a new article I may have a topic I want to explore, but in the end, it does not fit the journal I intended to submit it to. I can usually see that myself, but sometimes I find out in the peer-review process. This is especially true when I am writing about death and dying, my most favorite topic. As I have gotten older, my understanding of death and dying has been transformed and personalized by caring for my loved ones who have died. I have been known to add irrelevant (yet personally important) information about death and dying to articles. It happens; its human nature. Get help in the beginning, so the chances of successfully being published are higher. Be humble in the review process and trust experts in the field of editing. (See what not to do with your manuscript in Table 15.2.)

Another tip in understanding how others view your topic is to present at nursing conferences where you are not known. When you give a poster or podium presentation you will have a chance to give an overview of your project to others who are hearing about your work for the first time. Keep track of questions they ask. Address their questions in your manuscript in some way. Also make note of what others are presenting on a similar topic. Talk with those presenters about your topic and what they are doing. You may find people who have answers to questions you are proposing or who need your help in overcoming a clinical practice area. These conversations can be the start of a lifelong collaboration.

R = Record

Record all your thoughts on the topic, journal, author guidelines, and any communication with editors. Keep a folder on each journal you are considering. Your records for each journal should include:

1. Author guidelines
2. Editorial calendars/deadlines
3. Samples of articles that are similar in format to the type you think you may develop
4. Query letters and other communication with editors
5. Articles published by the journal directed at first-time authors; they all have them
6. Guidelines for becoming a peer reviewer
7. A copy of the manuscript you submitted, as one file and as separate files as required by the author guidelines
8. Peer-review comments
9. Revised manuscripts
10. Forms: copyright assignment, conflicts of interest, and others

Keep a list of possible journals to submit a manuscript to and the results of each submission. Only submit your article to one journal at a time. Be wary of predatory journals ("Beall's List," 2017). Track the peer-review comments you receive for your submissions. When comments relate to the readability of the manuscript, they are usually worth integrating into your manuscript. Some comments may be of limited value when they are addressing a niche topic that you have pursued in your DNP education or when they discuss topics like the use of technology. If you think the reviewers were not experts in important areas of your topic, appreciate their comments and volunteer efforts to help you develop your manuscript, but don't use the comments directly.

E = Enthusiasm

As you are preparing your manuscript, remember you are the primary cheerleader for it. You may need to "teach" others why you are so excited about your topic and project. Uncertainty about a new topic is not unusual. There are an unlimited number of subtopics within any general area in nursing; it is impossible to think an editor would have a working knowledge of every area of a given specialty. They don't have to be, that is what peer review is all about. The two to three peer reviewers will likely be subject matter experts and can give their feedback on the quality and accuracy of the manuscript to the editor. Let your enthusiasm show in your manuscript from the query letter to the reference list and tables. Don't let your manuscript become "homeless" when your enthusiasm fades (Fitzpatrick, 2017).

D = Dissemination

Dissemination via publication is the traditional method of sharing your scholarly work. Whether your work is a research study, quality improvement project, essay, or continuing education work, publication in a nursing journal is a very big deal and a success to cherish. Dissemination in a scholarly publication will require translation of an academic paper to meet the audience and formatting of the selected journal. There is no such thing as a paper done for class that directly translates to a publishable manuscript.

☐ Mechanics of Creating a Manuscript

Applications to Assist in Writing

There is a wide range of mobile and desktop applications that can also enhance the quality and decrease the time needed to compose a capstone paper. This book was composed using GoogleDocs, Dragon Naturally Speaking voice to text, and Grammarly to suggest edits to spelling and grammar. The final pages of the book were edited in Word.

Most universities provide deep discounts on the Microsoft suite of products. There are other options for word processing in addition to using Word. LibreOffice is a free option. However, it is not as powerful as Microsoft Word. If you are working from a template from a site, such as Smashwords or CreateSpace, Word can handle the headers and footers, as well as the page numbering. You can also use Google Drive or Microsoft's One Drive. Of the two, Google Drive offers the easiest options for creation of files and sharing.

If you're going this route, the best option for keeping your formatting intact is to export your document as a PDF. There are different options for exporting the document. At the very least, you want to make sure to embed the fonts. The print-on-demand site, Ingram Spark, requires PDFs be exported in the PDF/X-1a:2001.

There are several options that can streamline the writing process for you. Scrivener (https://www.literatureandlatte.com) is a popular choice for both nonfiction and fiction works. Although it is easy to learn, there are many nuances to the application for which you'll want to consult the user guide. I'm also including a link to its tutorials to walk you through the basics. This software recently released an Mac version of the program. Because of its interface and how it works with files, Scrivener may not be the best tool for collaboration if several people are working on the document at once. However, the advantage of Scrivener for these projects is that each chapter is created as its own file. With one master copy of the manuscript, others can work on other parts separately.

Voice-to-Text

There are specific voice-to-text programs. Dragon Naturally Speaking (Nuance) has always worked the best for me, but it does cost about $50 on sale. Windows 10 and OSX include speech recognition within their operating systems.

Grammar/Spell Check

There are several online and desktop options for editing. Some options are Hemingway, ProWriting Aid, and Expresso. Hemingway Editor is both a web-based tool and a desktop program. It checks for readability, adverb usage, language, and passive voice. It edits your work more for readability than grammar. The other two are more robust tools that check for additional metrics. Expresso looks at frequently used words, long sentences, filler words, and weak words, among other things. ProWriting Aid is the most robust tool, but is only necessary if you plan to make a career in writing. In addition to the basics, it scans for clichés, repeated phrases, transitions, homonym checks, plagiarism checks, and overused words. In this sense, it is most like an editor. Another nice thing about it is that you can use it with Google Docs.

Grammarly is both a free browser extension and a desktop app. As the name implies, it works with grammar rather than style. Because most of these applications offer free options, it certainly wouldn't hurt to run your manuscript through each one of them to see which is the best fit for an academic work. It's worth noting that ProWriting Aid allows you to select the type of text that is being reviewed.

Formatting for American Psychological Association Style and Other Formats

The Purdue Online Writing Lab provides an excellent source of all types of style guidelines, including citation guidelines. There are a number of tools for online citation assistance such as Citethis.com. There are also templates in all the major word-processing programs to guide you in the American Psychological Association (APA) style, which is commonly used in nursing. Use what is most convenient and simple for you.

Editing/Storing/Working in Groups

For editing, storing, and working in groups, Evernote, Box, and Dropbox provide good options for collaboration. All three allow you to enable two-step verification for extra security. They also offer mobile apps.

TABLE 15.2 What Not to Do With a Journal Manuscript

1	Submit to a journal if you have not followed the author guidelines
2	Submit to more than one journal at a time
3	Upload anything other than your very best work
4	Upload without the permission of coauthors or anyone mentioned in the acknowledgments section
5	Include anything copyrighted without permission of the copyright holder
6	Pay high fees for publication; the fees may not be listed in the author guides but they will be on the publication website; ask about any fees in the query letter to the editor before submitting your work
7	Submit your project paper, as is, to a journal
8	Not leave enough time to complete the follow-up that needs to be done once an article is going through the peer review process and post acceptance work

TABLE 15.3 Essentials of Submitting a Manuscript

1	Use applications like Grammarly to do an initial check of readability.
2	Use your university's editing services to improve readability; if this service is not available, consider hiring someone from a reputable agency. Many graduate offices have lists of reputable editors.
3	Use plagiarism-detection services and submit as a draft to double check any potential plagiarism issues before submission.
4	Write your manuscript as you go. Then make the selection of where the paper will be submitted early on so that the final version of the article takes a short amount of time to prepare because you will have followed the submission guidelines.
5	Sign up for the journal's e-Table of Contents to stay informed as to recent articles published in the journal; this is free. Better yet, subscribe to the journal.
6	Submit the reference list per the author guidelines; there are several types of formats often used; be sure to double check you are using the correct one.
7	Use your personal email when submitting. You may not hear back on the submission until after graduation and you may not be using your school-related email then.
8	If coauthoring a manuscript, one person will be designated as the corresponding author. Everyone should know the username and password for the account so that anyone can check the status of the manuscript.
9	Pay attention to detail. There are usually specific "conflict of interest" and copyright transfer forms that need to be completed before the submission can be peer reviewed.
10	Ask your employer or the organization where you completed your project for permission to use their name.
11	If you are asked to pay a nominal fee, and it fits with your purpose, consider doing this. Paying a nominal fee of $100 to $200 to allow nurses in countries who cannot afford access to nursing knowledge seems to be a reasonable request.

Reference Organizers

For a desktop solution, Zotero offers a standalone and web-based tool for storing citations. You can also store secure notes with it, making it a tool for collaboration as well. It is a citation manager so you can enter references and export a bibliography in the style of your choice. It includes numerous citation styles, including APA. It is free with limited storage. Another option is "Easy Bib," a web-based tool for storing and exporting citations. You can create separate bibliographies for different projects using MLA (Modern Language Association) or APA style. The *Chicago Manual of Style* style requires a paid subscription. The site is worth a look if just to research shared bibliographies and essay tools.

☐ Final Manuscript Preparation—Presubmission

As you reformat your university paper for publication, the journal's author guidelines are the essential document to guide you in the process. If you have a question not answered in the guidelines, send an email to the contact person (usually not the editor) listed in the guidelines. You will get an answer in a short time.

Before submitting the final paper, find a trusted person to read the article and give you a true critique. This person is not anyone you are related to, occupy the same residence with, or have an occupational relationship with. You want someone who is familiar with professional writing and will tell you the truth about the manuscript. If you don't know anyone, consider asking a university librarian to do it. Before we submitted our doctoral dissertation, we paid two university librarians to review the paper. One we asked to look at and double check our citations for accuracy and the second one to look at the format for understandability. They both did a great job for us. We specifically selected a librarian who was not familiar with our topic so that we would get questions from her that would reflect questions from readers who would be evaluating the paper and also did not know anything about the topic (Table 15.3).

Final questions to ask before submission:

- Is the manuscript formatted to the journal guidelines?
- Is this my best work?
- Have I removed all identifying information from the body of the manuscript?
- Do I have permission from all people and organizations mentioned in the article to use their names?

When you are ready to submit, this will most likely to be done electronically. You'll need to create an account at the publisher's page for the journal. Follow the steps listed. Generally the manuscript is divided into multiple files for blind peer review and there is a copyright release form you must sign and return before peer review can begin. It is a crucial step to follow the directions. Your manuscript will not be reviewed unless the directions are followed.

☐ Post acceptance Preparation

You should anticipate one final round of copy editing for any stylistic and technical errors. The deadline for this type of editing is generally a very tight.

It is essential that you are responsive to requests for this final edit. I'm always impressed with the efficiency with which copy editors review a publication. They always seem to find a small number of errors that were not caught by anybody else, including myself.

Caution, unless you have negotiated otherwise, you no longer have the copyright to your paper once it is published. You may be asked to become a peer reviewer in the submission or acceptance process. This is voluntary and your decision does not affect the acceptance or rejection of the paper.

☐ Ahead of Print

Once your article is finally approved and ready for print, it is likely to appear on the journal's website before the printed publication is available. Some journals have as long as a 1-year delay for the distribution of the print publication. And electronic publication ahead of print is always a convenient way to access your final product.

☐ Publishing a Book

Some may feel they have enough content and a unique point of view to create a book out of their DNP project. By all means look for a publisher! There are a number of sources for how to publish a book. Take a look at some of the most accomplished nurse writers. Consider contacting them directly. You may find a great mentor. Theresa Browne is one of the most highly regarded nurse writers with many books to her credit.

☐ Celebrating Publication

Once the publication is available, take time to celebrate this very important accomplishment. Very few people can say they have authored a publication of any type. Given all the work that you put into your project, it's very worthwhile to share it and celebrate with the people you love and who love you.

☐ Conclusions

Nursing science cannot grow and improve without people like yourself taking time to produce publications and presentations that inform the profession. It is entirely possible to get published in a professional journal in one type of column or another. With your passion and attention to the details of the publication process, it is a strong possibility that you will find your name in print one day.

REFERENCES

Beall's list of predatory journals and publishers. (2017). Retrieved from http://beallslist .weebly.com

Fitzpatrick, J. J. (2017). The homeless manuscript. *Nursing Education Perspectives, 38*(2), 56. doi:10.1097/01.NEP.0000000000000128

Kennedy, M. S., Newland, J. A., & Owens, J. K. (2016). Findings from the INANE survey on student papers submitted to nursing journals. *Journal of Professional Nursing, 33*(3), 175–183. doi:10.1016/j.profnurs.2016.09.001

CHAPTER 16

Speaking to Editors, Webmasters, and Practice Committees

☐ Chapter Checklist

☑	Speaking with editors
☑	Speaking geek with webmasters
☑	Speaking with practice and foundation committees

Throughout the process of completing your capstone project, you will be speaking to a number of individuals as well as representatives of various organizations and services. It is important to have a sense of the different types and methods used to communicate with specialists from all types of community organizations. This increases the chances of you being successful in acquiring the resources, access, and support for the projects you're involved in.

☐ Elevator Speech

Always assume that the person you're speaking with knows nothing about you, your topic, or your university. Always be mindful of the time constraints of other people and their potential lack of understanding of any specialized terms you use to describe your project. Perfect an "elevator speech." Elevator speeches are short explanations that are designed to engage the listener and concisely communicate the type and purpose of your project. A good elevator speech or pitch lasts no more than 30 seconds (Mindtools.com, 2017).

An example of an elevator speech used to publicize a press conference to announce the results of your community assessment project could be: "My project identified the top two concerns of voters in the community. I have valuable information on the issues and concerns of people who live and vote in this community." This type of description of your project engages the listener and leads to a natural call to action or invitation to events you are organizing around the project. Being honest, creative, and inspiring curiosity significantly increases the chance of individuals following your lead in making changes to the topic of concern and the people who are most committed to in your doctoral project.

☐ Headlines and Introductions

Editors are incredibly busy professionals who respond most effectively to concise and interesting proposals (Table 16.1). Starting your conversation with an elevator speech or engaging statement can make the difference in being able to describe your project fully or being turned away. Examples of headlines or invitations to talk about your project include:

- Give me 15 minutes and I'll save you 15 hours of frustration learning how to do (example).
- Can your readers recognize the seven early-warning signs of stroke?
- Will your readers benefit from knowing the 10 steps to stop smoking once and for all?
- Would you like to have an article on the best method for getting in shape after having children?

The key is to be confident, relaxed, make eye contact, and have a well-rehearsed simple and clear presentation for members of community organizations and publications that may be interested in knowing more about you and your project.

You could go one step further, especially for online publications, and check key terms that are being used in online searches. In order to find the key terms that are most likely to facilitate the new story being found in search engines, the process of search engine optimization is used. The first step in optimizing content going on the Internet is to identify the keywords that are collected by various applications online. One such popular application is buzzsumo .com. Use of these digital tools is what differentiates this text from others on dissemination. In Figure 16.1, you can see the results of a search for high blood pressure using BuzzSumo.

TABLE 16.1 Communicating with Editors

How to write a letter to the editor	www.virginia-organizing.org/speak-out-with-lte
How to write a query letter to a journal editor	www.writersdigest.com/online-editor/the-10-dos-and-donts-of-writing-a-query-letter
How to pitch an idea to a magazine editor	https://writersblock.loft.org/2013/10/25/2804/how_to_write_a_magazine_pitch
How to pitch a grant to a foundation committee	www.hewlett.org/friday-note-pitch-persuasive-or-how-to-maybe-get-a-grant

FIGURE 16.1 BuzzSumo results for key-word search.

☐ Webmasters

Occasionally, you may have the need to speak with a webmaster about content on a webpage that exists or to suggest content you would like to see added. Webmasters are generally not content experts in the material included on the webpages that they maintain. However, they are keenly interested in ensuring the content is accurate and current. The time I most often contact the webmaster is when I see an inaccurate citation or a broken link to something that's on his or her page. Sending a comment about something that needs to be corrected on a web page is a positive communication in the eyes of a good webmaster.

TABLE 16.2 Communicating With Webmasters

Google webmaster blog	https://webmasters.googleblog.com/2016/03/best-practices-for-bloggers-reviewing.html
How to speak geek	www.zdnet.com/article/how-to-speak-geek-and-influence-nerds-wait-what
What does a webmaster do	www.youtube.com/watch?v=s6AD0AN42vw
Free webmaster help	www.freewebmasterhelp.com

Communicating with the webmaster is similar to communicating with other content managers. Generally speaking, there will not be a phone number to use to call the person who manages the web page. Instead, there will be a link to an online comment box or an email address. You may or may not obtain an answer to your correction or comment. However, you can check back with the web page to see whether your suggestions have been incorporated into the content.

Webmasters can be influenced to add content by your expertise in an area, although he or she may not be the only individual with the authority to add such content. Look for the link to submit content ideas. If it is not clear, find the webmaster contact information and send an email asking for the link.

☐ Communicating With Practice Committees

All of the communication suggestions I've been giving so far have focused on one-to-one communication. There may be opportunities for you to present your ideas to groups of people or committees that have the potential to approve your project, fund your project, or participate in a broader application of changes suggested by your project. These are very exciting opportunities, and your passion and expertise in the topic should be evident.

Presentations to groups of people are usually highly structured with tight timelines. Many, for example, may meet only once or twice a year at regular intervals. In order to understand what is expected of you when you are communicating with a group of individuals who have met for a specific purpose, you can ask for any written guidelines, review a website, complete a web search on past activities of the committee, and check their social media profiles.

The more prepared and informed you can be on the mission and purpose of the committee, the greater the chance of you being successful with your requests. Like other forms of specialized communication, it is suggested that you lead with a concise elevator speech and finish with a call to action that describes the specific response you would like from the group. Always leave time for questions so that members of the committee can obtain additional information from you. Always leave a business card and written proposal or request at each meeting.

☐ Conclusions

As people get to know you and learn more about your efforts to implement some type of practice change to better the lives of a group of individuals, they may provide additional opportunities for you to give presentations to influencers and decision makers in your community. Every opportunity to add value to a website, a forum, community organization, or other agency that shares your goals should be looked at as a golden opportunity to improve the quality of life of the people around you.

REFERENCE

Mind Tools. (2017). Crafting an elevator pitch. Retrieved from https://www.mindtools.com/pages/article/elevator-pitch.htm

CHAPTER 17

Initial Submission of Work

☐ Chapter Checklist

☑	Prepare one document for archiving.
☑	Did you follow author guidelines?
☑	Separate components of the article for individual upload.
☑	Assess an electronically generated review copy of the manuscript.
☑	Monitor review activity electronically.
☑	Ancillary documents required for review (copyright releases)

Submitting your manuscript for consideration as a potential publication in a peer-reviewed journal is a big step. It requires a tremendous amount of hard work and persistence to produce a manuscript. Submitting the product of your doctoral program not only leads to an evaluation of your writing skill but also your ability to describe and professionally present all of the learning you underwent in the program. It is no small impact.

☐ Preparing the Manuscript for Submission

It is important to follow the author guidelines exactly as they are described when submitting the manuscript for the peer-review process. An excellent resource

TABLE 17.1 Preparing the Manuscript for Submission

1	Keep the complete file with all components of the manuscript in a folder.
2	Separate individual parts of the article as directed in the author guidelines.
3	Ensure that the title page is the only part of the submission that gives identifying information for the author or authors.
4	Label tables and figures in individual documents and direct the editors about the placement of the tables and figures within the body of the article.
5	Ensure the file names of each part of the article are clear and accurate.
6	Check the electronically prepared consolidated document once the submission is complete for accuracy. Re upload any files that need to be replaced before submitting for review.

from the notes authority Heather Carter-Templeton (2015) provides additional information on the process of converting a capstone paper into a publication. In general, the steps for submitting an article are described in Table 17.1. Most submissions will be fully electronic, which allows you to track the progress of the article through the review process. You will be able to log on to the publisher's review system any time you would like an update on the progress of the review. Failure to follow the process described in the journal author guidelines is one of the more common reasons for rejection and delays in reviewing (Kennedy, Conwell, Newland, Owens, & Pierson, 2015).

Peer Reviews

The peer reviewers for your article will also be using the electronic management system to conduct their reviews. As a result, you will be able to see how many reviewers were used and their progress in reviewing the document. You will not be able to see their comments until the editor of the journal reviews the comments and makes an initial determination on whether the article is appropriate for publocation, based on the editor's and the peer reviewers' comments.

Occasionally, you may be asked to submit names of potential peer reviewers of your manuscript if the topic is highly specialized. You should give the editor names only when asked. The editor will contact the people you suggest for a formal discussion of the process.

Revisions

The need to revise the manuscript after peer review is almost a given. Whether the reviews are minor or major, the electronic system tracks each action done to the manuscript. A document may need to be revised several times before a final acceptance is obtained. As individual files related to the article are edited, it is important to have the most current version of files clearly labeled, ensuring the correct, edited documents, are uploaded accurately and in a timely way.

If any errors occur in the process, it is important to notify the editor immediately. Errors do occur and the publisher may need to issue a correction in future journal publications should they occur. With diligence and persistence a few, if any, corrections will need to be issued. The goal is always for a document to be completely accurate at the time of publication.

☐ Ancillary Documents

Publishers will also require that one or more ancillary documents be submitted along with the manuscript. Generally speaking, there are two that will be needed in order for the article to be reviewed. The first is a release of copyright, which indicates that once the article is accepted for publication the author no longer holds copyright to the work. There are a growing number of exceptions to this in which the author retains the copyright after publication.

Some journals are "open access" and allow authors to maintain the rights to their intellectual property. Many of these journals are reputable; however, some are considered predatory. You can determine which type of journal you are submitting your article to by referring to Beall's list of predatory journals.

The second document that is required as a separate file or an online assessment is a statement of any potential conflicts of interest. Authors must disclose any relationship they have with products or services mentioned in the article or any money received from vendors, grants, or other financial incentives they may have received related to the subject of the manuscript.

☐ Conclusions

The electronic submission of your article is an exciting activity that signals you are nearly at the end of a long journey. Accuracy and diligence in the process ensure that the correct documents are reviewed and the publisher is assured that submissions meet a common set of ethical standards for honesty and lack of bias due to conflicts of interest.

Electronic submission systems allow authors to track the progress of their manuscript at will. Although the process is highly technical, it is still a deeply personal experience. The submission of the manuscript is an important developmental milestone in your lifelong journey as a professional.

REFERENCES

Carter-Templeton, H. (2015). Converting a DNP scholarly project into a manuscript. *Nurse Author & Editor, 25*(10), 2. Retrieved from http://naepub.com/student-authorship/2015-25-1-2

Kennedy, S., Cowell, J., Newland, J., Owens, J. K., & Pierson, C. (2015). *Findings from the INANE member survey on student papers submitted to nursing journals.* Paper presented at the July INANE conference Las Vegas, NV. Retrieved from https://inane2015.files.wordpress .com/2015/07/inane-member-survey-on-student-papers_final_july-20-2015.pdf

CHAPTER 18

Rejection and Revisions

☐ Chapter Checklist

☑	What a rejection means
☑	Managing revisions
☑	Developing a professional thick skin

Receiving a peer review that asks for many revisions or results in a rejection can be difficult. These experiences are part of a lifelong path of disseminating information. There are reasons that a rejection may occur that are within your control, some that are out of your control, and some that could have been prevented. Following the author guidelines and asking questions if you have them are two important ways of navigating the world of publishing. What is important to know is that rejection happens to absolutely everyone at some point during one's career. Like rejections, revisions are an integral part of the peer-review publishing process. Because the reviews are blind, there is nothing to take personally because no one who interacted with the manuscript knows who you are.

Some excellent suggestions for handling rejection are found in an article by Laursen (2009), "If at First You Don't Succeed, Cool Off, Revise, and Submit Again." Laursen suggests cooling off before responding to a rejection. The same is true for revision request. As the author, you have two options when responding to the rejection. If you get comments from the editor, you can revise your paper and resubmit. Or you can submit the article to another journal. Most of the time

TABLE 18.1 **Steps to Take Following a Manuscript Rejection**	
1	Take a deep breath and relax before doing anything.
2	Take time to review the editor and reviewers' comments and reflect on their accuracy.
3	Don't give up.
4	Contact the editor with any questions about the comments.
5	Edit the manuscript using the peer-reviewer comments as a guide; it is not always necessary to comply with the request for revisions. Most editors will take the comments under advisement and rely on you to argue the merits, or lack thereof, of reviewer's comments.
6	Revise the article to comply with any guidelines mandated by the journal.
7	Keep a record of your submission activity, including accuracy of peer-reviewer comments, timely responses from the editor, and other important aspects of the submission process for each journal.

changing the publication means revising the manuscript in some way (Table 18.1). Depending on the reason for rejection, you may want to consider a read/write of the manuscript. Some flaws are fatal for manuscript such as lack of novelty or uniqueness (Ali, 2010).

☐ Requests for Revisions

If you are asked to make revisions, it is important to decide in a timely way whether you will address them or not. It is entirely within your right to decline to make any or all revisions to a manuscript and let the editor determine whether the comments were important enough to result in a full rejection of the manuscript. Editors do have discretion when it comes to peer-reviewer comments, which are meant to advise the editor on the manuscript's worthiness for publication. The editor has more knowledge of what the readership wants from the publication and may request a different set of modifications be made in order to publish the manuscript. It is rare that an editor would contradict peer reviewers but it may happen with a well-reasoned argument from an author who disagrees with the peer-review comments. Provenzale (2010) gives a lot of useful advice in handling requests for revisions, including what happens when reviewers give opposing comments—a suggestion to keep in mind is to disagree without being disagreeable.

☐ Conclusions

Handling rejection and suggestions for revisions are part of the development of a thick-skinned professional. They are a part of the process experienced by all people on the journey to becoming a published author. Some reasons for rejection or requests for revisions are well within the author's control, such as compliance with the author guidelines. Some are not under the author's control, for example, when a manuscript is rejected because it is similar to an article already in process. The point is to not be discouraged and give up with your first rejection. There are many more journals to consider for resubmission by continuously perfecting your knowledge and insight about the publication process; there is a journal waiting to publish your paper.

REFERENCES

Ali, J. (2010). Manuscript rejection: Causes and remedies. *Journal of Young Pharmacists, 2*(1), 3–6. doi:10.4103/0975-1483.62205

Laursen, L. (2008, August 15). If at first you don't succeed, cool off, revise, and submit again. *Science.* Retrieved from http:// www.sciencemag.org/careers/2008/08/ if-first-you-dont-succeed-cool-revise-and-submit-again

Provenzale, J. L. (2010). Revising a manuscript: Ten principles to guide success for publication. *American Journal of Roentgenology, 195*(6), W382–W387.

CHAPTER 19

Acceptance and Follow-Up

☐ Chapter Checklist

☑	What a rejection means.
☑	Managing revisions.
☑	Developing a professional thick skin.

When you receive notification that your article has been accepted and is scheduled for publication, celebrate first. Then realize the work is not over. You will need to complete the revisions discussed in the last two chapters. You will need to respond to other members of the publishing staff who may request further edits related to the quality of the copy and readability of the content. Timeliness is an important aspect of developing your skills as a writer. Even though an article may not appear online or in print for several months, there is still urgency in responding to any requests made by the editor or publisher.

☐ Responsibilities After Acceptance

In addition to responding to requests from the editor and publisher, there are few additional activities you can take the lead in to help ensure the success of your publication. Publicizing the acceptance is a first step in making sure the article is seen by others. Make conference presentations on the content in your article in order to promote it. Volunteer to be interviewed on podcasts or by bloggers to gain additional exposure for your article.

Another way to promote your published work is to create a short video or publication trailer, somewhat like a movie trailer, to use in social media. You can also create an introductory slide presentation and upload it to SlideShare or graphic (see Chapter 11) to pin in Pinterest. You can also create hyperlinks to the journal or publisher to help people find the whole publication. You cannot send full text files of the article because you generally do not own the copyright after it is published. Ask the editor about any questions you may have regarding copyright restrictions.

☐ Tracking the Impact

In addition to seeing your name in print, impact on nursing practice is the highest goal of sharing your work. Informing nursing practice can be measured by tracking citations through online databases. You can also use Google Scholar to track access and articles that use your citation that in future publications. You can also create a Google Alert in order to be notified of mentions of your keywords, which are somewhat similar to hashtags; citations and discussions that appear in social media, in classrooms, and at professional meetings.

If you find a need to correct anything in the article after it has been published, be proactive and let the editor know immediately upon finding out about the error. A correction will be published at the first opportunity online and in print. If the correction is significant, the entire article may be retracted.

☐ Retractions of Published Articles

Retractions of published articles are a very rare event. If you are interested in knowing more about how an article gets retracted and what is done to the author of articles that have been retracted, you will find a wealth of information on the blog, Retraction Watch (retractionwatch.com). This website provides a unique and valuable service to consumers of research by bringing together a wide range of information on scientific misconduct and fraud.

Notable for new authors is a case study of what happens when a scientist's findings cannot be replicated by others and an error is discovered. Such was the case with Pamela Ronald and Benjamin Schwessinger (McCook, 2015), who were completely transparent about their inaccurate results when it was found there were errors in an original report of theirs due to no fault of the authors

As the author of a published manuscript, you are in charge of ensuring it is not only accurate at the time of publication; you should continuously monitor its accuracy by following the trail of utilization that may occur as a result of publication of a well-written and timely paper.

People make errors, usually through not following the steps outlined in the SHARED model. Keeping accurate records of where you got your information and other resources is essential to being able to trace your work, should there be a question in the future. It is not realistic to think you can remember everything you did related to your manuscript development; notes are important if there is a question in the future. The key is to respond immediately to inquiries about sources. If you cannot find the necessary information in your notes, use the Wayback Machine (archive.org/web) or an Internet archive.

☐ Conclusions

At times, it is may seem like an author's work is never done. The post acceptance work needed to assist in final edits, publicity, and ongoing vigilance about the article are well worth the rewards (nonmonetary) for having the rare opportunity to say you are a published author. Your article is like anything else you have created. It has your signature, your values, and interests all over it. You and you alone could have produced it (or your group). Take care of it.

REFERENCE

McCook, A. (2015). What do you do after painful retractions? Q&A with Pamela Ronald and Benjamin Schwessinger. Retrieved from http://retractionwatch.com/2015/07/24/qa-with-pamela-ronald-redemption-after-retraction

CHAPTER 20

Podium Presentation to Professionals: Conferences, Posters

☐ Chapter Checklist

☑	SHARED model
☑	Completing proposal
☑	Acceptance of proposal
☑	Preparing presentation and poster
☑	Engaging with the audience

A professional presentation begins many months before the actual presentation. Plan far in advance of the conference at which you hope to present your project as the call for presentation proposals usually occurs many months in advance of the event. This is your time to shine. You will be among your colleagues—those you know and have yet to meet. Many other doctoral students will be given poster and podium presentations on their projects. Follow the steps in this chapter to complete the process to have your accepted proposal ready for a podium presentation. Like publishing, the acceptance of a presentation proposal is the first step. The invitation to give a presentation is an honor. Sharing what you know, is something special and unique to you, for all to hear.

☐ SHARED Model

S = Select

Selecting your topic for a presentation begins with the familiarizing yourself with the specifications of the conference proposal. Every conference has a theme. Some are very specific such as pediatric surgery care. Others are more general such as nursing education. Regardless of the topic, you must modify your work to fit the themes of the conference, its format, and timeline of the presentation.

The most difficult guideline to follow in developing a proposal is to select the most relevant content that can be professionally presented in 15 minutes, which is the most common time limit for research/project presentations. This means you will take only a small portion of your work for presentation.

H = Habits

The habits you will need to develop or enhance concern being concise, relevant, and professional. You may also need to develop some technical skills to use technology available at the conference. If your proposal is accepted, reading about what to expect at the conference is key to making sure you are well prepared for your presentation. Other habits to develop include gaining skill with presentation slides, fostering audience involvement, and managing questions from the audience. Audience questions may get you off track or cause you to run overtime. It is necessary to be professional and polite in order to stay on track.

A = Assess

Assessing your skills in developing a presentation, giving the presentation, and managing the audience are important. All these skills require practice.

R = Record

Recording drafts of the proposal, conferences you would like to attend, and developing timelines are essential when presenting at a conference. When submitting the proposal you may be asked if you have a preference for giving a poster or podium presentation. You can indicate your preference or declare you have no preference.

E = Enthusiasm

Remaining enthusiastic is perhaps the most essential part of preparing and giving your presentation. People are deeply affected when a speaker is passionate about the topic.

D = Dissemination

Disseminating a presentation is an honor and something to approach with the same scholarship as a print publication. Giving a presentation at a nursing conference is helpful if you plan to publish your presentation. You will get valuable insight into areas of your ideas that are not clear by noting questions from the audience.

☐ Completing the Proposal

Each conference will specify the types of presentations requested. Often the conference will have a theme and specific categories of work they are looking for. Follow the proposal guidelines exactly as requested. If you are doing a presentation that involves any special equipment be sure to ask the conference organizer whether it is possible to use the equipment during your presentation. Like a publication, make sure everyone listed on the proposal has given permission and will be in attendance at the presentation. Many conferences ask you to specify whether you want to give a poster or podium presentation. Both are excellent ways to present your work. In my experience, presenting a poster provides a much greater opportunity to talk with people directly about your work. Podium presentations are generally 15 to 30 minutes long, which is not a lot of time to present a project that took you 1 to 2 years to complete. The choice is yours. Speak with your advisor about the best choice for you (Table 20.1).

Central to your proposal is communicating the essence of you project. How you do this is your choice. Reading from slides is not the answer. Consider using few words and more visuals. Seriously consider what the audience wants to know before completing your proposal. Your capstone document is written for your faculty, yourself, and regulators to show that you mastered certain competencies.

TABLE 20.1 Tips for Preparing Conference Proposals

Tips on conference proposals	http://blog.tesol.org/tips-on-writing-successful-conference-presentation-proposals
Conference proposal checklist	http://scottberkun.com/2011/speakers-checklist
Sample conference proposals	www.cgu.edu/pages/919.asp
Center for Innovation in Research and Teaching	cirt.gcu.edu/research/developmentresources/research_ready/presentationready/powerpointpresent

The conference is going to choose whether to have you or someone else presenting. Make sure your proposal shows your passion for the topic.

Submit the proposal on time and wait for the conference organizer's determination of acceptance. In the meantime, continue to give the presentation to anyone who will listen and perfect your presentation skills. It is also helpful to create a poster that matches the requirements of the conference you are hoping to attend. You do not need to print anything, rather you can upload the material to your own website if the conference does not have one. You can give people the link to a site where they can find handouts. There are many websites to explore that can help you design an engaging scientific poster presentation. Find one that is easy to use and start making posters for various aspects of your poster presentation for different audiences. As you create the slides for your podium presentation and poster, be sure to get permission to use school and other agency logos and names.

After you have been accepted, be sure to confirm your acceptance and attendance at the conference. If you find you are unable to make the conference, be sure to let the organizers know. You will usually need to register (at the student rate) in order to be included in the program. Often there is a discount for presenters, but conferences are rarely free. This is a very unfortunate aspect of doing presentations.

As you develop the proposal, create the presentation, and review evaluation comments, consider the needs and expectations of your audience. At nursing conferences, consider how many people in the audience will be students, faculty, and clinicians. There is likely to be a mix of all three. If the audience is likely to be composed mainly of students, consider their level of study. Also, consider whether they are attending your presentation for course credit or if they have an interest in the topic. Understanding the expectations of the audience will help you understand how to develop your presentation.

Developing presentation skills begins by immersing yourself in presentations made by others. TED (Technology, Entertainment, Design) talks are among the best. Table 20.2 lists an example of some interesting nurse-related TED talks. There is a big difference between a project presentation and a keynote speech. Start small when giving public presentations. Present the material to the staff on your unit first. Offer to give presentations to different students in your nursing program. Ask for anonymous feedback to promote authentic comments. Take note of questions you are asked at practice presentations and include them in the content for your conference proposal.

Creating the slides or handout for your presentation should follow some simple guidelines. These are:

1. Less is more—Highlight keywords, simple colors, and use one or two fonts.
2. Maintain consistency with the same colors you will be using to promote your message in the future.
3. Use visuals; stock photos are available but photos you took are best.
4. Find examples of slide presentations at SlideShare.com.

TABLE 20.2 **Nurse-Related TED Talks**

	Title	Link
1	Atul Gawande: How Do We Heal Medicine?	www.ted.com/talks/atul_gawande _how_do_we_heal_medicine
2	Carolyn Jones: A Tribute to Nurses	www.ted.com/talks/carolyn_jones _a_tribute_to_nurses?utm_source =tedcomshare&utm_mediumreferral &utm_campaign=tedspread
3	B. J. Miller: What Matters at the End of Life	www.ted.com/talks/bj_miller_what _really_matters_at_the_end_of_life
4	Alice Rawsthorn: Pirates, Nurses, and Other Rebel Designers	www.ted.com/talks/alice _rawsthorn_pirates_nurses_and _other_rebel_designers
5	Sarah Gray: How My Son's Short Life Made a Lasting Impression	www.ted.com/talks/sarah_gray _how_my_son_s_short_life_made_a _lasting_difference
6	Peter van Manen: Better Baby Care—Thanks to Formula 1	www.ted.com/talks/peter_van _manen_how_can_formula_1_racing _help_babies
7	Mary McKenna: What Do We Do When Antibiotics Don't Work Anymore?	www.ted.com/talks/maryn _mckenna_what_do_we_do_when _antibiotics_don_t_work_any_more
8	Myriam Sidibe: The Simple Power of Handwashing	www.ted.com/talks/myriam_sidibe _the_simple_power_of_hand_washing
9	Jennifer Brea: What Happens When You Have a Disease Doctors Can't Diagnose	www.ted.com/talks/jen_brea _what_happens_when_you_have_a _disease_doctors_can_t_diagnose

☐ Podium Presentation

Developing Good Presentation Habits

As you are developing your presentation skills, seek out models of good presentation. Once again, look at TED talks, they are the best 15 (or so)-minute presentations. There are ample resources at the TED site to help you develop a presentation. The habits and skills needed to give a presentation include a clear focus delivered in

EXHIBIT 20.1 **Principles of Good Photography**

1. Keep the images relevant to the topic.

2. Use emotionally powerful images when necessary.

3. Use the rule of thirds to place elements in the frame. Divide the frame into 3 rows and 3 columns to place the subject in the proper location (Photography Mad, n.d.)

4. Make sure you have permission to use images of people.

the form of a story. The presentation material should be simple and provocative. There are many nursing presentations at TED.com.

Most presentations are supplemented with slides of some kind. Typically, there are six to eight slides used in a short speech. The slides usually include the following:

- Title
- Objectives
- Review
- Acknowledgments
- References

Consider that people may have access to the slides long after you have made your presentation. Make sure the content stands on its own and your contact information is available on them. There are many resources to help you design a powerful set of slides to supplement your presentation. A familiar site, the Purdue OWL APA resource, also has information on formatting a presentation with excellent examples (owl.english.purdue.edu/owl/resource/686/03). Check the website newdnp.com for additional examples. To include photographs, follow the simple photograph guidelines listed in Exhibit 20.1.

In the Microsoft-owned website SlideShare.net, there is a section on "Editors Picks" that includes some of the best slide presentations uploaded. Take a look through the SlideShare depository and get inspired to create your own template. Throughout the process of defining your topic, style, and message, continue to refine your colors, images, and metaphors you use. Once you have a good set of slides, you can do a lot of things with the slides. If you want to produce an eBook, you can sit down in front of the computer with the slides and record your presentation. That recording can be turned into a transcript. That transcript can become a book. The slides can also be saved as jpg files and used in a video you create as title and transition slides.

The presentation often needs to be sent to the conference organizers well in advance of the actual presentation. Once you have submitted it to be uploaded to the conference technology team, do not make any additional changes to it. Stay focus on the content that was accepted by the review committee.

Giving the Presentation

It goes without saying that you must arrive on time and be ready to give your presentation. Being ready means that you have practiced and don't require the slides to read your presentation. Instead, you will use them as a backdrop to your content. Have your business cards ready and a backup of your files available if giving a podium presentation. The Write-Out-Loud.com website is full of very helpful information on giving presentations. If you need help in overcoming the fear of public speaking, you can attend meetings of Toastmasters International (www.toastmasters.org) to help you become the best presenter possible. If using posters you may need to bring the thumbtacks or other materials to use to attach the poster to the wall or board that will be used to showcase the work. The posters are generally assigned to a specific location, so be sure to check in with the organizers so that you place your poster in the right location.

☐ Audience Engagement

Regardless of how short your time allotted is, involve the audience (Table 20.3). Have the audience move in some way. Using your objective(s) as a guide, select a portion of your work that is most likely to be of interest to the audience and fit the time frame you have been given. Every second you go over your time limit is time lost to the next presenter.

Straightforwardness is an important skill to incorporate into your presentation. There isn't enough time to have a complicated warm up at a scientific conference. Ensure your content is relevant to the majority of the audience. It's impossible to be relevant to everyone in the audience. Make your best estimate and verify your plan with the conference organizer.

TABLE 20.3 Interactivity for Presentations

1	Storytelling techniques	www.sparkol.com/engage/8-classic-storytelling-techniques-for-engaging-presentations
2	Storytelling techniques training	http://blog.langevin.com/blog/2012/04/02/10-best-practices-for-using-storytelling-in-training
3	Social media	https://www.forbes.com/sites/work-in-progress/2014/01/28/five-easy-tricks-to-make-your-presentation-interactive/&refURL=&referrer=#66db0433976a
4	How to use props in presentations	http://scottberkun.com/2011/speakers-checklist
5	Tips for making presentations interactive	www.ncsl.org/legislators-staff/legislative-staff/legislative-staff-coordinating-committee/tips-for-making-effective-powerpoint-presentations.aspx

Even though it will be a scientific conference, you can still use humor that does not demean anyone else. Pick something to make light of, perhaps something that is familiar to members of the audience. An exemplar of humor to use is the work of comic illustrator Randy Glasbergen. Randy is an internationally known cartoonist and creator of many comics, called simply Glasbergen. His health and medical related comics are well known (http://www.glasbergen.com/diet-health-fitnessmedical). Comics related to the subject of your presentation can engage the audience and leave them with a positive feeling about your topic. Always ask permission for anything you use. Even when the resource is "free," consider making a small donation to the creator to offset the costs for providing the service. At least leave a review on the website to help them with their rankings on the Internet.

The most important recommendation I can make is to practice, practice, practice. Record yourself and review the recordings. Watch the expert presenters who give the TED talks and review their suggestions for making presentations. It is especially important to practice if you are going to use props of any kind. Visual aids are very effective in conveying ideas and bringing information alive. They can bring clarity and credibility. Dr. Oz is expert in using props on his show. Perhaps you can watch him do this. The props must complement your metaphors and other design items you have previously used.

☐ Posters

There are many resources for creating professional-looking posters. Take the time to develop a poster that shows your best work and reflects who you are as a professional. A 3-foot by 4-foot poster can cost as little as $20 to $30 to make. Many universities will assist in the development of the poster and provide it for free. Some universities have a template for the poster, be sure to use this if there is one.

Poster presentations that are a collection of 8 × 10 pieces of paper pinned to a board do not represent the level of achievement that a doctoral degree represents. There are many new advances in the creation of posters. Given the templates at printers, there should not be any need to hire a graphic designer for your first poster presentation. Rather, you should assemble a synthesis of core material from your project along with images that support that your content. You can use the colors of your brand to further identify the poster as part of your professional activity.

Posters used to be very difficult to transport as they often were mounted on foam board and were large flat pieces of paper that needed protection in transport. Later posters that could be laminated and rolled up were popular and remain so. A new advance in posters that I've enjoyed using is printing the poster on cloth. The poster is folded up like any other object and placed in your suitcase. These posters cost approximately $200 each, so they may not be the type of poster you would want for your first experience presenting a poster because of the cost. Consult with your faculty advisor and personnel at your work to see whether there are extra funds available to finance the purchase of a poster and travel expenses to present the poster. Like all other uses of a logo or other images, it is necessary to obtain permission to use any logo or copyrighted material on a poster, even though it is for educational purposes.

☐ Storytelling

Consider your oral or poster presentation as a story with a beginning, a middle, and an end. Storytelling is not new, yet its effectiveness in conveying information and engaging the audience is hard to beat. Whether you are using slides, sophisticated digital media, or simply standing at a podium, storytelling works. People love to meet heroes, take the journey with key characters, be surprised and moved by the people in your project. Ask to have photos of memorable people and relate experiences that occurred during your project, even if you have not completed the project yet.

There is no presentation that can include the entire timeline and list of activities involved in your project. You must be selective about what to include and what to eliminate. That is what good storytellers do; they are conscious of what makes a good story that engages the audience. They leave off material that may be meaningful to them, but is not meaningful to the audience. They take the time to bring audience members along on the difficult and joyful portions of the story.

☐ Conclusions

There are many techniques that can be used to make a presentation interesting, engaging, and relevant. The key is clarity and focusing on the main message, and then integrating stories, props, and other innovative content to make your project memorable.

REFERENCE

Photography Mad. (n.d.). Rule of thirds. Retrieved from www.photographymad.com/pages/view/rule-of-thirds

CHAPTER 21

Presentations to Lay/Community Audiences

☐ Chapter Checklist

☑	Develop an oral presentation for the lay public
☑	Target your audience
☑	Storytelling basics
☑	Publicity campaigns for your projects

All presentations need to be adapted to the audience that will be in attendance. Creating an engaging presentation for nonhealth care professionals can be one of the most fun types of presentations to give. Providing a quality presentation for the lay audiences who were the focus of your project is an important part of showing respect to the individuals who supported you through the process of completing your project.

☐ Developing the Presentation

Once you have completed the project, select the most relevant information for the lay people in the audience. They will want to know about results and what they mean to the individual, rather than the methodology you used to produce the project. In other words, the opposite of what the faculty is looking for in your defense of the project. Presenting a clear message that highlights your core message is the most important decision you make in planning any presentation.

The second most important decision is the method used for presentation. Third, develop a creative and interesting presentation that the audience will remember. You will not be able to describe everything about your project. You will want to be highly selective about what you present to others; always be careful to plan your presentation based on what your audience wants to hear.

A very interesting context for the development of an engaging presentation was presented by Takashi Iba (2014), a transdisciplinary researcher, creator, and writer, in "Presentation Patterns: A Pattern Language for Creative Presentations." He has contributed to the field of research in creativity. I summarize his main components in the next section. Iba believes a creative presentation is imaginative, thought-provoking, portrays the presenter's feelings, and engages the audience. Creative presentations are not just an explanation but a creation; they do just teaching, rather they help students to make discoveries. The central idea is that there are three main presentation patterns (and an additional 30+ subpatterns) in a creative presentation (Iba, 2014). There is an excellent SlideShare presentation on his ideas available at www.slideshare.net/takashiiba/pattern-language-30-and -fundamental-behavioral-properties-takashi-ibapurplsoc15-keynote-2015.

Types of Presentation Patterns

The Main Message—Identify the most important message and build the presentation around it in a way that best conveys that message. This component incorporates the primary content as well as the best communication process— storytelling, drama, and so on.

A Touching Gift—The presentation is a gift for an audience. They may understand the message but are they moved to share your feelings? Here is where you focus on who *they* are, what they think about, and how you can gain their sympathy. Additional presentation techniques as well as audience participation ideas come into play here.

Image of Success—The presenter sets a clear goal for the audience to achieve. This image is kept in mind when creating the presentation as well as actually presenting it. Because there are many ways to present information and inspire action, it is critical to stay focused and on track with your message.

Every Presentation Is a Story

Regardless of the type of presentation you are giving, it should have a beginning, middle, and end. Describe your purpose simply and engage your audience quickly with a story, humor, images, music, or any other method that evokes some type of emotion or active engagement (Anderson, 2016). Watch Dr. Oz or *The Doctors* TV show to see how they craft messages in a few minutes between commercials for the general public. Entertainment is an important part of all presentations, but especially for the public that does not have an in-depth knowledge of your topic. Often audience members will have a specific goal in mend when attending your presentation—to learn more about a favorite topic, to become advocates for your cause, to help you raise money, or many other possibilities. End every presentation with a call to action. Leave the audience with suggestions for an action they can take to make a difference.

Importance of Audience Engagement

There is almost a limitless number of ways to include the audience in your presentation, irrespective of its length. Interaction is key to keeping their interest and making the content memorable. Here are some suggestions:

Let people know how you will handle questions, how to contact you at the end of the presentation, and express gratitude for their time. Find a way to interact with the audience throughout your presentation. Make them partners in the information. Have them share with each other, with you.

Include some type of assessment activity that is interactive. Consider asking the audience to stand while doing some initial activities. Other assessment activities may include asking the audience members to interact with each other or to complete a short web-based questionnaire. Or present a concept and then, rather than using the raising of hands to indicate agreement, have audience members move to different portions of the room based on their stance on the issue. Consider the time needed to move people around in the planning of your presentation. Precious time can be lost when asking audience members to move around the room. If the activity is really engaging, the time is worth it. However, deliberate instruction for returning to their seats or remaining where they are is needed to stay on time.

Games, such as quizzes, question and answer, twenty questions, and other game-show formats—such as *Jeopardy* or *Who Wants to Be Millionaire*—are great ways to check understanding of content when giving a presentation. If a game is going to be effective, it needs to relate to significant information and reinforce attitudes that are important to the audience members' job success. They also should "be enjoyable and engaging without being overly simplistic or silly."

Ask for interaction: Tell the audience you expect interaction from the very beginning and have designated times to encourage it. In this digital age, incorporate use of smartphones to respond to survey questions or tweet feedback.

☐ TED Talks

The exemplar of scientific, artful, short video presentations are seen in the worldwide phenomenon of TED (Technology, Entertainment, and Design) talks (www.ted.com/talks). There are thousands of TED talks online in every subject imaginable. Certainly the advent of TED and TEDx has revolutionized how we engage and convey information and content. We are all familiar with this approach: The presentations are brief, they are delivered without notes (requiring much scripting and rehearsal), and they are "professionally visualized" (well-crafted audiovisulas, good props, and good lighting). Yet these elements don't really get to the heart of the effectiveness of TED talks.TED talks owe their effectiveness to a few points (www.scienceofpeople.com/ted):

1. TED-style talks are personal. You give such a talk about something that you are passionate about and that passion is felt by the audience.
2. TED talks can take the audience on a journey.
3. TED talks are short. And because of that, there are no extraneous words, rambling rabbit holes, or irrelevant points or information.

So the concepts of personal passion, going on a journey, and delivering a focused message are key techniques to take from TED talks to apply to any presentation (Karia, 2014).

Once you have created your script and have practiced the content, it can be given via an in-person presentation, radio, podcasts, television, multimedia, or any other presentation method. An excellent presentation always begins with a well-planned, well-rehearsed program that is presented in a natural way. If you need to add some creativity to a presentation, consider the methods listed in Table 21.1.

TABLE 21.1 Resources for Creating the Script for a Lay Presentation

Resource	Location
Lisa B. Marshall's Public Speaking Podcasts	There is a list of the 12 most popular podcasts at www.lisabmarshall.com/publicspeaker
Toastmasters International—an organization dedicated to assisting individual to become excellent public speakers	www.toastmasters.org
How to give a TED talk	www.ted.com/about/conferences/speaking-at-ted
Tips for writing a presentation script	www.free-power-point-templates.com/articles/tips-for-writing-a-great-presentation-script
Presentation script—check you word-processing program for a template	www.template.net/business/outline-templates/presentation-outline-template

Here are a number of other findings from my research into creative presentations:

1. Incorporate music, memes, or a dance ensemble: Enlist a volunteer and create and act out a scene that illustrates your points.
2. Pay a makeup artist to make you look like a very old man/woman and present as if you came from the future and are telling people what will happen.
3. Create a mood board in real time or engage your audience in doing it. Have a number of objects and samples and text relevant to the topic and allow audience members select items to add to the collage.
4. Make a painting.
5. Make a mind map in real time as you tell your story or weave your presentation.
6. Create a flash mob.

☐ Hashtags

Hashtags are short combinations of characters that identify an event; created for Twitter, they are widely used in social media. Choose a hashtag early in your project and use it throughout the project any time you post on social media. You will need a Twitter account to be able to post content with hashtags. Twitter is heavily used by reporters. I would give up all my other social media accounts and keep Twitter if I was only allowed to have one! The hashtag used for this text is #NEWDNP.

Before, during, and after presentations, you can use the hashtag to collect comments about your work. You can also do a large amount of your publicity for community and other presentations through social media using hashtags because often journalists only take story leads generated through social media.

Anything you print out should include your hashtag. You can also create alerts in Google to be notified via email if the hashtag is used.

☐ Publicity

It will often be necessary for you to be involved in publicizing presentations you will be giving on your topic. Even if you are not asked to get involved, consider volunteering to be involved so you can be sure that the people you are most focused on are aware of your presentation. Keeping a list of people you have contacted and have helped you complete your project is a good place to start when publicizing anything you will be doing to get the word out about your project. Developing an email list is a great way to keep supporters and others up to date with what you are doing. After that, local newspapers, radio stations, TV, bloggers, and podcasters are great contacts for your press releases.

FIGURE 21.1 **Sample press release.**

Contact Information:

[Company/Individual] social media info: Hashtags, pages

[Email, phone, social media usernames "@Twitter"]

[Name and/or description of event]

FOR IMMEDIATE RELEASE

[City, State] – [Company/Individual] will present [Name of Event], taking place at [Location of Event] on [Date], and featuring a presentation on an important community topic related to health [describe an interesting part of presentation].

[Company/Individual] invites all interested members of the community to [Name of Event] at [Location of Event] to become informed about how this issue affects the health of our community. [Name of Event] will [further description on what will take place at event].

[More details about event; cost, or need to RSVP]. Always say something about parking in an urban area.

Press Releases

Press releases are announcements of important information and events. There are many templates for press releases available online. Figure 21.1 includes one I have used many times.

Press Conferences

It may be necessary to plan a press conference or other media event in order to get the best turnout for your presentation. This is especially true if you are working with a small organization. Creating a publicity campaign and planning a press conference are very similar to planning a nursing meeting.

How to Conduct a Publicity Campaign

Initial Planning

Craft your message and know the outcome you want to achieve. Gather together the stakeholders in your project and determine the message that is most important to share with the public. List your main points and set outcomes you can measure for the dissemination presentation.

Once the goals are identified, list the types of news agencies and specific reporters who cover this type of information. Include not only names and specialties, but also their social media memberships. Follow them early on and assess what they are interested in. You can offer follow-up to stories they are publishing. Find them on Twitter, Instagram, Facebook, and other social media. Allow time to contact the media representatives you want to attend. Many news organizations prefer messages in social media to traditional paper or faxed press releases. But you may find you will need to do some cold calls to inform reporters about the event. Friday evenings are excellent times to make cold calls.

Create an online home to publicize your event. A Facebook event page is free and has many features that will help guide you through publicizing the event. Use your branding colors, images, metaphors, and other reusable objects you have created on the Facebook Banner. Canva (Canva.com) is a great free tool with many templates to create Facebook headers and many other graphics.

Press Conferences

Have printed information available in the room for the conference. Ensure members of the press are welcomed and sign in or are admitted into the conference once they are introduced to the organizers. Have your contact information and business cards available. Make sure you have clarified whether what you are presenting represents your employer or your own effort. If you are using your employer's name, you will need permission.

There will be times when there will be more than one presenter and you will need to offer information on each person who is presenting, including names, titles, contact information, and roles in the project.

SMART Techniques

The essence of your message works best when it is positive and shows your project's benefit to the population, community, and systems that are included in your project. Begin by making a calendar that includes all your events. Include other deadlines such as proposal guidelines and graduation deadlines (Table 21.2).

Public Statements

Making public statements can take a number of forms. In-person conferences are the most traditional, but streaming services in social media such as Facebook

TABLE 21.2 SMART Goals for Press Conferences

S	Specific—Focus on one or two important priorities.
M	Measurable—Make action steps something that can be easily evaluated.
A	Achievable—Frst steps are something that can be accomplished.
R	Relevant—Address the needs of those involved in the project.
T	Timely—Create a timeline that is acceptable, clear, and takes into consideration everyone's ability to meet deadlines.

or YouTube are also excellent ways to disseminate publicity about your project and the results of your project. See Table 21.2 for SMART objectives for press conferences.

The best public statements, tweets, or other social media content have a focus, something new and interesting offered in a few words that could be a headline. Include links to your web page or contact information, so others can find more information on the topic. Make your content interesting to the press or subscribers by including photographs, links, multimedia, or other engaging content.

Take the time to notice who is writing and announcing specific topics in your community. Read their columns; subscribe to their blogs, social media channels, or other content. When you speak with them, ensure you relate your project content to their existing efforts. Let them know you are aware of their interests. Your contributions will help them do their jobs better. Don't be shy; reach out when you see articles on similar topics. Reporters and bloggers may be most interested in developing expertise on topics they have already presented. The new content needs to be presented in interesting ways.

☐ Conclusions

There are many techniques that can be used to make a presentation to the public interesting, engaging, and relevant. The key is clarity and focus on the main message, and then integrating stories, props, drama, and other visual aids to bring the message alive for the audience.

REFERENCES

Anderson, C. (2016). *TED talks: The official TED guide to public speaking.* New York, NY: Houghton Mifflin Harcourt.

Iba, T. (2014). *Presentation patterns: A pattern language for creative presentations.* Yokohama, Japan: CreativeShift Lab.

Karia, A. (2014). *TED talks storytelling: 23 storytelling techniques from the best TED talks.* Publisher: Author.

CHAPTER 22

Multimedia: Videos, Photographs, and Online Repositories

☐ Chapter Checklist

☑	SHARED model
☑	Planning multimedia—assembling individual components
☑	Basic design principles
☑	Storing virtual presentations

Creating multimedia presentations can be one of the most fun and interesting parts of your dissemination plan. There are many excellent examples of user-generated videos on YouTube and many educational sites. You can do all of the creation from your mobile device. Videos are popular. They should be fewer than 3 minutes long and engaging. By using the resources included in this text, you will be able to maintain the intellectual property rights of others by using copyright-free resources. It is also necessary for you to indicate what copyright licenses you are going to withhold or give to other users who may be interested in repurposing and using your own creations.

☐ SHARED Model

S = Select

Select the topic from your project that you will present using multimedia. Multimedia presentations are generally fewer than 15 minutes. If you have a topic that cannot be reduced to 15 minutes, split the topic into individual parts.

H = Habits

Habits that need to be developed include planning presentations that are focused on the topic; are concise; and developing scripts, slide presentations, and audio recordings. Each will be discussed in this chapter.

A = Assess

Assess what you know already and how your video will add value to your message.

R = Record

Record the progress you make and the software and hardware tools you use. Especially track copyright permissions, authorship of material, and technical specifications for hosting your media online. YouTube, Facebook, Instagram, and iTunes or Stitcher all have different requirements for hosting content. Most have little to no associated costs. However, some projects and material will be very popular and could have additional hosting expenses.

E = Enthusiasm

There are several technical skills you need to develop to produce a multimedia project. They are all doable and are skills well worth learning. If you find your enthusiasm decreasing due to dealing with the technology, reconsider the scope and depth of the project. Nothing is more important than the message. Make sure the content remains the most important part of the media. Ensure that all the images, colors, music, and other content support the message.

D = Disseminate

Dissemination via a video is a timely way to share your project with others. Many tools are available to create a video for YouTube, Facebook pages, or other social media. Disseminating short videos—as short as a minute—has the potential to introduce your project to people around the world. Creation of a video can be done

FIGURE 22.1 **Storyboard.**

Title of Project		Date:	
Version #:	Name:	Contact:	
Slide #1	Slide #2	Slide #3	
Script	Script	Script	
Slide #4	Slide #5	Slide #6	
Script	Script	Script	
Slide #7	Slide #8	Slide #9	
Script	Script	Script	

with any smartphone. Careful planning is necessary to be effective. A storyboard is the equivalent of an outline for a paper. No matter how brief your video, plan carefully.

☐ Planning Multimedia

Most of the material you developed for your project will be the basis of your storyboard or outline in that it includes descriptions of images, video, and other content you will use. Storyboards are essential to ensuring your presentation follows your topic (Table 22.1). There are many resources for creating storyboards online. The storyboard is a screenshot-by-screenshot description of the video image, script or text, sounds, and action. Carefully planning even a one minute video improves the quality. Having a complete storyboard also makes it easier to edit as necessary.

TABLE 22.1 **Resources for Creating Videos**

1	Storyboards	www.storyboardthat.com
2	Tips on using a mobile device for video recording in three easy steps	www.cyberlink.com/learning/video/67/create-videos-on-a-mobile-device-in-3-simple-steps
3	Applications for editing videos created on mobile devices	iMovie (Apple) Magisto Android
4	Directories to upload video content on the Internet	YouTube Vimeo
5	Animation XTRANORMAL White Bear	Examples: www.youtube.com/watch?v=pwUCw0vi1zY&list=PLX9rPXD2bm_a5e0PRymTro3nr3AoEtkDa www.youtube.com/watch?v=6MaSTM769Gk&list=PL09D747AA6ACDFF71
6	Applications GoAnimate NAWAL for Schools	goanimate.com www.nawmal.com/schools
7	Explainer videos Animaker	www.animaker.com

As you begin to consider how you will present your project, there are several different ways to create the video. A straight presentation with a beginning, middle, and end is the most common. Another way to create a video is to follow the process of creating an unfolding case study ("An Unfolding Case Study," 2017).

An unfolding case study leaves room to request audience participation, even if the presentation is done asynchronously online. You can also provide information over several issues of a video. Another type of presentation can be a video with alternate endings in which you can create two different conclusions for a case study presented in the introductory video. The principles of creating alternate-ending videos are described by Robertson (2013).

☐ Creating Multimedia

Creating multimedia begins with a solid plan that operationalizes the objectives of your project and uses appropriate images, text, references, and other video. The creation of any multimedia begins with the completion of a storyboard or outline of how the file will be created. Once the storyboard is complete, any number of programs can be used to edit video that is recorded on your mobile device.

It is most helpful to create a detailed slide presentation, not one that will be given to the public, but one that includes all your important information. Then the content from the slides can be transposed to the storyboard.

Mobile Phones

All you need to create a video is in your mobile device. You can create a video by using your mobile phone to record the action. A few apps can improve the final product, such as screen shares.

Animation

Animation is also an interesting method to use to convey information. An exemplar of animation is the now defunct service Extra Normal. Although users are no longer able to create their own videos, a number of extraordinary videos exist on the web as examples of simple, yet effective content. A second exemplar is the polar bear series (www.youtube.com/watch?v=6 -MaSTM769Gk &list=PL09D747AA6ACDFF71) in which relatively sophisticated cartoons are used to depict the trials and tribulations of the life of the polar bear. This funny and entertaining series is included in order to inspire you to consider using a similar service to deliver your message. Animation, or cartoons, are commonly effective for children and young adolescents; however, they still have a place in the education of adults as you can see from both of the series referenced here.

Explainer Videos

Explainer videos are a relatively new resource to use in educating consumers, staff, or others about a specific topic. A typical explainer video is 30 to 60 seconds long. They are new, so their novelty increases the chance of them being viewed. There are many existing tools to create your own explainer video and services that will create them for you.

☐ Other Interactive Multimedia

Games, including quizzes, game shows such as *Jeopardy*, or many other templates assist in the creation of educational games and quizzes. *Who Wants to Be Millionaire* is a game that can be fun and engaging. If a game is going to be effective, it needs to relate to significant information and reinforce attitudes that are seen as important to the audience members' understanding of the topic. Games also should be relevant, engaging, and focused. The basic criteria for creating online games and quizzes are described in Table 22.2. Several studies support the use of educational gaming in health care education (Boyce, 2016; Rojas, Kapralos, & Dubrowski, 2016; Woodson, Jones, & Timm, 2012).

☐ Conclusions

Designing contemporary digital and online teaching tools provides some of the best methods of both disseminating and reinforcing the most important messages of your project. You can upload links and embed or upload to your own blog or website in order to keep all your educational resources in one place.

REFERENCES

An unfolding case study (Ideas for Engagement series). (2017). Open SUNY COTE. Retrieved from https://www.youtube.com/watch?v=LFvclHApcd4

Boyce, L. M. (2016). Play it, learn it, make it last: Developing an online game to create self-sufficient library information users. *Medical Reference Services Quarterly, 35*(3), 274–284. doi:10.1080/02763869.2016.1189781

Robertson, M. (2013). How to let viewers choose an ending to your interactive video [Creator's Tip #80] Retrieved from http://tubularinsights.com/viewers-choose-interactive-video-creators-tip-80

Rojas, D., Kapralos, B., & Dubrowski, A. (2016). The role of game elements in online learning within health professions education. *Studies in Health Technology & Informatics, 220*, 329–334.

Woodson, D., Jones, D., & Timm, D. F. (2012). Playing online interactive games for health education: Evaluating their effectiveness. *Journal of Hospital Librarianship, 12*(4), 351–362. doi:10.1080/15323269.2012.719191

CHAPTER 23

Blogs

☐ Chapter Checklist

☑	Introduction to blogs
☑	Choosing a hosting platform
☑	Using templates
☑	Budgeting time
☑	Copyright permissions—giving and receiving

Blogs are one of the most exciting parts of the Internet. Blogs are web-based platforms that experts, individuals with an opinion, corporations, and many others generously give of their time and talent to educate, inform, and entertain people with similar interests. There are blogs that are essentially black holes of negativity, but these are the exception to the rule. I could live the rest of my life without television, but not without the blogs I follow and enjoy. They have made my life richer and more meaningful.

Blogs are also a tremendous amount of work. I maintain three, more or less, and I greatly admire the individuals who are able to maintain a consistent presence and provide valuable content. For the purposes of a blog that you may maintain for your capstone project, you need look no further than the exemplar website of ProBlogger.com. I will be mentioning other blogs but this particular blog is without a doubt one of the highest quality websites, full of the richest possible free content you can imagine. Many blogs are complemented by other social media resources

TABLE 23.1 **Basic Blog Pages**

Landing/home page	First page seen by visitors to your blog
Blog	Page where all postings will appear in chrono-logical order with newest first
About me	Page that describes who you are and what the purpose of the blog is
Contact	Describes how to contact the blogger; consider getting a Google Voice phone number so you do not have to use your personal phone

and podcasts. ProBlogger is one of those; the founder, Darren Rowse, has spared no expense of money or time to provide this exceptional resource.

☐ Why Blog?

The biggest advantage of starting a blog is that you can collect all of your essential information in one place (Table 23.1). A blog would allow you the opportunity to collect email addresses, lot surveys, to post content, and provide links to other valuable information related to your topic. WordPress is the most common blog platform in the United States. It has a robust support community and many sources of templates, help documents, and examples of best practices.

It is not necessary to be a computer programmer or geek to have your own blog. Templates provide all the setup structure you need to begin blogging within just 1 or 2 hours of signing up for WordPress. Many free templates for blogs, using different color combinations and themes, are freely available. It is not necessary to spend much money on a blog. I do recommend you obtain the URL for your name and any keywords relevant to your topic. You do not need to use them, but maintaining them costs around $20/year and is worth the investment.

☐ How to Create a Simple Blog

To begin creating a simple blog, you will need to first sign up for a WordPress account, download a template for blogs, and design the site to match your project colors and other graphic design components you have decided on. It is important to place a professional headshot of yourself on the home or landing page. There is a free version of WordPress that is more than adequate for your dissemination project.

TABLE 23.2 Best Free Blog Templates

Activello	https://colorlib.com/wp/themes/activello
News Maxx Lite	https://wordpress.org/themes/news-maxx-lite
Freenity	https://wordpress.org/themes/freenity

TABLE 23.3 Examples of Quality Blogs

500 Successful Blogs	www.sparringmind.com/successful-blogs
Best Nursing Blogs	www.toprntobsn.com/50-top-nursing-blogs-for-2015
Particularly Good Nursing Blog	https://thenerdynurse.com
Donna Cardillo, RN	https://donnacardillo.com
The Nursing Show	www.nursingshow.com

The typical pages on a blog include:

- Landing or home page
- Blog postings, with categories for searching
- About me page
- Contact page

Many free templates are available specifically for blogs (Table 23.2). A simple Google search will produce a large number of possible templates. Be sure to pick one that is described as "responsive," meaning it is formatted for mobile devices. Table 23.3 lists some blogs with quality content relevant to nurses.

☐ Copyright

Advanced practice nurses are very familiar with copyright and the requirements for proper citation of sources. Refer to your university library for additional information. What many students don't realize is that it is necessary to consider the copyright restrictions or permissions you are giving others to use your work. The Creative Commons Foundation (https://creativecommons.org) has done pioneering work in the area of promoting open access to intellectual property. Through their advocacy, you can look for specific "licenses" on web content that proactively informs the user as to what she or he can and cannot do with information on the website.

Take the time to indicate to visitors to your website or blog what they can do with your material. Almost everything on the Internet is to be considered copyrighted unless the copyright has expired, it is specific governmental reports, and other material. Ask the contact name at the source what the permission is if it is not clear.

Be aware that more and more copyrighted material can be used for educational purposes. See Appendix 2 for a comprehensive list of websites with freely available photographs and artwork. Of course, every single item used requires a citation. Image resources are necessary because every blog post should include some type of image or graphic. You can make it yourself or use one of the resources listed in Appendix 2.

☐ Resources for Following Blogs

Before you decide to create a blog, start reading them. There are several applications you can use to collect and read them in one place. I don't recommend signing up for them to be delivered to your email. Your inbox will soon be overrun with postings. Feedly is my favorite aggregator. I read blogs as I have time and generally skim them once or top twice throughout the day. Setting up Google News searches using keywords from your project will provide you with an ongoing and consistent source of new information related to topics of your interest. Setting up Feedly (https://feedly.com) to collect information on topics of interest to me is a small investment of time as I have gained hundreds of hours in time saved by being spared the need to search in a traditional library. (I have shared my feeds: https://feedly.com/newdnp). As I find the material I want to use for future publications, blogs, or other uses, I can automatically save postings from all of my Feedly feeds to Evernote (Table 23.4).

Aggregating blogs in a service like Feedly also makes sharing content to other social media platforms very simple and effective. By combining Feedly with another free service Hootsuite, I am able to share blog postings to Pinterest, Twitter, Facebook, LinkedIn, and Google Plus. I know I have become a more informed professional, citizen, and athlete as a result of the generosity

TABLE 23.4 **Resources to Enrich Blogs**

Feedly, blog aggregator	http://feedly.com
Hootsuite, social media aggregator	http://hootsuite.com
Buzzsumo, keyword search database	http://buzzsumo.com

of content creators for the blogs I follow and the ease with which I am able to synthesize large amounts of data with little effort and time investment.

Blog postings contain the following:

- Images
- Engaging headlines
- Content with links;the more content the better
- A short bio at the end of every posting
- Categories, tags, and keywords, so users can search for prior postings on topics
- Hyperlinks to contacts and other online resources you are discussing
- Links to social sharing to media such as Facebook, Instagram, and others
- Hashtags are included for key content

Web-Friendly Content

Creating Images

In addition to stock images or photographs you have taken, you can create engaging images that incorporate your project design elements with a free tool: Canva (http://canva.com). Canva is the graphic design application of choice. You can also embed video and live stream webinars to a blog.

Conclusions

Blogs are the simplest way to have a web presence. Resist any temptation to purchase programming or other services that you probably don't need for this level of blog. Instead, concentrate on becoming familiar with online writing techniques and format related to blogging by following exemplars. As you progress toward the completion of your project, you can use the blog as a source to store links, references, and other resources that will be of benefit to you and the people you serve in your project. Blogs are proof that people are generous, kind, and very willing to help strangers in a time of need. You can repay the generosity of people who educated you through their blogs by linking back to the sources you used from their websites. That is the ultimate "thank you" on the Internet.

CHAPTER 24

Using Your Talents and Interests to Do Something Innovative

☐ Chapter Checklist

☑	Assess your talents to find where your heart and mind meet.
☑	Be brave; step outside your comfort zone.
☑	Advocate for yourself and your ideas when they are rejected.
☑	Don't give up when you meet the first barrier.

You will probably do a capstone project only once in your life. As a result of this unique experience, you have a rare opportunity to take charge of the process and make a truly meaningful contribution to nursing science. You can do this by selecting a topic that is on the cutting edge and critically necessary for the quality of life of the people you are assisting. These people may or may not be well known to the larger community; their problems may be invisible to others, and solutions nonexistent. Your topic may have to do with geriatric orphans (people who have outlived all their family members), undocumented immigrants, victims of sex trafficking, or those with developmental disabilities who live in group homes in your community.

The greatest doctoral project, or I should say my all-time favorite, is the Beads of Courage program (www.beadsofcourage.org) founded by Dr. Jean Baruch, who saw a need for children with cancer to be recognized for the intense treatment they had undergone. One nurse took it upon herself to develop a local program

TABLE 24.1 Nurses Who Have Inventions

1	Lorraine Parthemore invented the Parthemore Pulley for orthopedics	www.stuff.co.nz/taranaki-daily-news/news/10489453/Neck-pulley-reaches-Innovation-finals
2	Sister Jean Ward (1950s) developed the bilirubin light used for neonatal phototherapy Adda M. Allen designed the baby bottle containing an internal liner	www.mcknights.com/the-real-nurse-jackie/a-nurse-invented-that-but-most-likely-didnt-get-credit-for-it/article/374465
3	Joyce Harrell, RN, OCN	Adds a table to every type of pole. http://traybl.com
4	LinkedIn Nurse Inventor Group	www.linkedin.com/groups/3838150/profile
5	*Independent Inventors Handbook*	www.amazon.com/dp/0761149473
6	Resource for Innovations	Basic information for inventors: http://edisonnationmedical.com

that has grown into an international program that brings together community members who are interested in supporting children with cancer and their families by giving money or beads at their local hospital with a program to the main organization to be given to children with cancer. All of us have the potential to develop a program for some issue or group of people in our communities (Table 24.1).

The unique contribution that this book makes in helping readers develop 21st-century digital skills is to provide a launch pad for advanced practice nurses who are committed to changing the world by improving the lives of patients and their families and communities. This is no small job. But you can do it; you have made the first giant step toward changing the world. By considering disseminating your project via social media, you have given the world access to your ideas. Many more people may be moved by your work than if it only appeared in a scholarly journal seen by very few people.

☐ Suggestions for Personalizing Your Ideas

You may decide to "brand" your ideas with a unique way of presenting the information, for example, by creating a coloring book. Adults now routinely enjoy coloring books as a way of learning and relaxing. Another idea might be to create a mobile application that highlights your area of experience and resources. Simple

TABLE 24.2 **Playlist of Stress-Relieving Songs for Student Nurses**

	Song Title	Artist
1	"Every Storm Runs Out Rain"	Gary Allan
2	"I'm Movin' On"	Rascal Flatts
3	"Bless the Broken Road"	Rascal Flatts
4	"Broken Windshield View"	Chris Lane
5	"Nobody's Perfect"	Miley Cyrus
6	"Only Human"	Jason Mraz
7	"I Will Survive"	Gloria Gaynor
8	"My Heart Will Go On"	Céline Dion
9	"I'm No Stranger to the Rain"	Keith Whitley
10	"I Won't Back Down"	Tom Petty
11	"Meet in the Middle"	Diamond Rio
12	"Lean on Me"	Bill Withers

card games, word puzzles, or make-believe experiences can highlight a topic from how to promote customer service to providing end-of-life care.

You can also focus on specific multimedia, such as creating a playlist, to underscore your message (Table 24.2).

☐ Conclusions

The doctoral program you will be completing is just the beginning of constructing fences to prevent or minimize the suffering of others through your daily work and the project you have completed in your program. Just think of the changes you have already made, not only in your own life, but also in the lives of others, and this is just the beginning.

CHAPTER 25

Disseminating an Artful Scholarly Project

☐ Chapter Checklist

✓	Using art to deliver your message
✓	Screenplays
✓	Music
✓	Poetry
✓	Responding to critiques of your work

Using art to disseminate information about your project magnetizes the audience and creates a special opportunity to make the content memorable. The two exemplars of this are the journalist and nurse advocate Suzanne Gordon (Gordon, Hayes, & Reeves, 2013), who used a table reading of scripts to focus on enhancing teamwork and communication. The script is pure genius and a truly novel way to bring home the message of patient safety. A second example is seen in the actress well known as Nurse Jackie's boss, Anna Deavere Smith, in her one-woman show, "Let Me Down Easy." These are both highly experienced people with a passion. This chapter is about helping you find a different way to present your information that both entertains and informs.

Step outside your comfort zone to disseminate your work. Do something no one expects or maybe something people think you cannot do. If you show your enthusiasm for the topic by going all in, your audience will appreciate the effort. Table 25.1 lists some innovative ways to present health care topics.

TABLE 25.1 Screenplays of Health Information

Let Me Down Easy by Anna Deavere Smith	www.youtube.com/watch?v=uQ1OyKy9FwM
Suzanne Gordon, Lisa Hayes, Scott Reeves	Bedside Manners: Play and Workbook (The Culture and Politics of Health Care Work)
Nurse's Day Show—Operation Theater	www.youtube.com/watch?v=BToz2hlH_5o
If We Could See Inside Others' Hearts	www.youtube.com/watch?v=Wl2_knlv_xw&index=16&list=PLD0955F38770CB49C
Pink Glove Dance	www.youtube.com/watch?v=cTylhMLp3FA
From Crisis to Drama	www.youtube.com/watch?v=CFmBU3WtOAo
Selves Portrait—A Senior Thesis Portraying Schizophrenia Through Dance	www.youtube.com/watch?v=KnHnbmOzZTo

☐ Using Art to Deliver Your Message

Performances

Acting out the results of your project can be one of the most rewarding ways of delivering your message. It may seem unlikely to consider such a choice but I encourage you to consider the possibility. Creating a short performance can instantly put the audience in touch with the emotions and message of your hard work.

Once you have composed your project document, you have the material to write a short screenplay. There are free tools to help you, such as Plotbot (www.plotbot.com). Google Docs also has a screenplay template available (http://bit.ly/2bgH2El).

Music

> *Music is the electrical soil in which the spirit lives, thinks, and invents.*
>
> —Ludwig van Beethoven

Music has the power to transform lives and to bring hope and comfort to people in challenging circumstances. There are many free sources of music to use in disseminating your project (Table 25.2). Choosing the right music to include in a presentation or to create yourself varies according to your objectives. Bluegrass and jazz may be preferred in one area of the country while natural

TABLE 25.2 Resources to Assist with Creating Musical Presentations

Title	Source
Incompetech	http://incompetech.com/music/royalty-free
Moby Gratis	www.mobygratis.com
ccMixter	http://ccmixter.org
Partners in Rhyme	www.partnersinrhyme.com
Musopen	https://musopen.org
Public Domain 4U	http://publicdomain4u.com

sounds or classical music may work best in other areas, but all cultures have musical preferences.

Music is relevant at every stage of life. However, its effectiveness can vary in different life stages as well as from patient to patient. The clinical use of music is now an evidence-based practice that has been proven both to satisfy patients and, very significant, to lower the cost of care.

Music has also been shown to enhance the experience of patients waiting for well visits—it improves individual awareness of the hospital, enhances the speed and efficacy of staff performance in surgery, and even ameliorates the anxiety of patients being weaned from mechanical ventilation. Music has the potential to minimize the procedural and environmental demands that the conditions of the intensive care unit place on patients, and it can engage and help to retain typically elusive patient groups in areas such as mental health and substance abuse. In addition, music has the potential to encourage people to commit to routine and necessary preventive care. If you would like to include music and are not a musician, ask a local musician to accompany you during the presentation.

What type of music is best for which audience? The delivery of music that is "appropriate" in health care settings is more than an issue of satisfying a generic checklist of do's and don'ts. The brain of each individual patient has picked up musical building blocks from the local sonic environment in infancy and developed preferences based on that experience. To the extent possible, music needs to resonate with the message you are sending about your project. Ideally, music should be relevant to its listeners in terms of culture, genre, mood, and era of origin.

The use of music in health care is being transformed by technology. Already, technology is used to offer relaxation and entertainment, enabling listeners to

TABLE 25.3 Playlist of Songs About Death

	Artist	Song
1	Kathy Mattea	"Where Have You Been?"
2	Kathy Mattea	"That's the Deal"
3	Elton John	"The Last Song"
4	Martina McBride	"I'm Gonna Love You Through It"
5	Bomshel	"Fight Like a Girl"
6	Tim McGraw	"Live Like You Were Dying"
7	Rascal Flatts	"Skin"
8	Death Cab for Cutie	"What Sarah Said"
9	Simple Plan	"Save You"
10	Rascal Flatts	"Stand"
11	Ben Folds Five	"Hospital Song"
12	Cold War Kids	"Hospital Beds"
13	Craig Morgan	"Tough"
14	Anthony Phillips	"Bleak House"
15	Tim McGraw	"Don't Take the Girl"
16	Joey + Rory	"When I'm Gone"
17	B.B. King	"See That My Grave Is Kept Clean"
18	Elvis Presley	"Long Black Limousine"

TABLE 25.4 Poetry to Enhance a Presentation

1	Amy Gerstler	*Medicine* (collection of poems)
2	Dylan Thomas	"Do Not Go Gentle Into That Good Night"
3	Maya Angelou	"When Great Trees Fall"
4	John Donne	"Holy Sonnets X"

access and respond emotionally to a subject. Music can be used as the introductory sound people hear and the final sound that is heard during a presentation or class. Because so many adolescents already record and sample music, technology can also provide an avenue of influence with this age group.

Use songs that resonate with your message. Consider offering a playlist of music that supports your message. Table 25.3 contains a playlist of songs about a peaceful death that I use often before, during, and after presentations.

Poetry

The use of concise and well-placed poems can move the audience and set the tone for your presentation (Table 25.4). The Poetry Foundation (www.poetryfoundation .org) has a huge repository of poems for all occasions.

☐ Responding to Critiques of Your Work

Even the best presentations receive negative feedback of some type. Because a performance may be more personal than other methods of dissemination, it may be a challenge to respond to a "bad review." Some reviews will not warrant a comment, if they are personal in nature.

You are also likely to get positive and encouraging critiques of your work ("What to Do When People Criticize Your Art," 2017). Most people want to encourage risk-takers. But that is not always the case. If you encounter people who have negative criticism about your art or performance, there are a few steps you can take to cope with the bad evaluation. First and foremost, if the person does not know you personally, don't take what they say personally. Stop yourself from doing or saying anything. Instead, take a deep breath before responding. Think before you speak. Don't feel obligated to listen to all the comments. However, obtaining feedback is important and essential. Instead of receiving real time feedback, ask for feedback via paper questionnaires or online. Make it easy to obtain the feedback and be *brief.*

The Media

Opinions by the local media may be solicited or unsolicited. If the feedback is negative, the primary goal is to stay calm—there is nothing to be gained from letting your hurt or anger get the best of you. Next, try to keep an open mind. Is the source credible? Does this person know what he or she is talking about? Perhaps he or she makes a good point. It is unlikely that these critics will know you personally and it is very important to remember not to take their words personally. Again, objectivity is key when evaluating feedback. No response is necessary to media reviews that are negative.

☐ Conclusion

Use your creativity to develop a dissemination project that does not just inform people who are interested in your topic, but also entertains them. A screenplay can evoke emotions and enhance the ability of the audience to recall the essence of your topic many years in the future. Step outside your comfort zone and do something new.

REFERENCES

Gordon, S., Hayes, L., & Reeves, S. (2013). *Bedside manners: Play and workbook* (The Culture and Politics of Health Care Work). Ithaca, NY: ILR Press.

What to do when people criticize your art. (2017). Retrieved from http://www.artbusiness.com/artists-how-to-evaluate-and-respond-when-people-criticize-your-art.html

CHAPTER 26

The First Dissemination of Your Work Is the Hardest

☐ Chapter Checklist

☑	Preparing for your presentation
☑	Professionalism in presentations
☑	Photographs in presentations
☑	Translating complex information to different audiences
☑	Involving the audience
☑	Archiving the presentation

Presenting your work, especially for introverts who have never spoken in front of an audience, can be very challenging. You are likely to be giving presentations to both your university and the agency where you did the work. You may also be presenting the results to the participants in your work, such as the community group who participated, or members of the media, such as television or newspaper reporters. Take every opportunity you can to tell others about your work. Refer to Chapters 3, 10, 18, and 21 for assistance in developing general speaking skills. Review the information in Unit IV for creating presentation material.

As you plan each of your presentations, do so with the understanding that no one knows you or the topic. Even if you know every single person in the room and all of them are familiar with your topic, you should begin at the beginning of your topic and proceed to the end as if you and your topic are unknown to the audience. You can include audience members in different ways during the presentation if they know you or the topic. Ensure each presentation stands on its own merit and is complete. (See Exhibit 26.1 for a presentation transcript.)

☐ Presentation Preparation

The most important rule of presentations is to know your audience. The second rule is to know what is expected of you. The third rule is don't bore anyone. You are there to educate, translate technical information so it is understandable to anyone, and entertain the audience so that they will remember what you said. *That means your presentations should be visual, short, and include audience participation.* No matter how brief a period of time you have been given and the number of people you will be speaking to, with planning and practice you can produce a memorable presentation.

Knowing the Audience

You may be giving the same core content of information to different groups of people. The board of directors of your hospital is a very different group than the clinical staff or community members who are interested in your topic. Review any written material you find on the purpose of the group of people you are presenting to. There is a wealth of information on agency websites, self-studies for accreditation, newspaper articles, and biographies of notable people in the audience. Make it your business to find out all you can before speaking to a group. If possible, attend a meeting of the group before you give your presentation. If it's not possible to attend a group meeting, ask to see minutes of meetings or other documents related to the working of the group.

Professionalism in a Presentation

When you are developing your presentation for each audience, do so with a commitment to being professional. By professional I mean use no humor that marginalizes any group, no images that are irrelevant and could be considered "cheesy" or don't add to the strength of the presentation and are placed just to entertain yourself and a few people who know you well.

Likewise, when you give the presentation your dress must be consistent with the dress code of the organization that invited you. You may have a polo shirt with a university logo on it for more casual presentations, such as those delivered in an outdoor location or to a community organization focused more on leisure activities. Otherwise, wearing professional attire, not a scrubs uniform, is essential attire. You can augment the presentation by coordinating the colors you are wearing with the colors of your brand. If you have received clothing gifts from the people you have worked with, be sure to wear them if appropriate.

A clever way of dressing for a large meeting occurred at an academic meeting at an online university. The president gave a 20-minute presentation on the state of the university. In between his presentation, awards were given in various categories. He introduced various members of the administrative team to give the presentations. In between his introductions, he changed shirts. He changed into shirts that various departments in the university had given him. It was a wonderful way to connect with a very large crowd. It was a memorable presentation that I will never forget. Once again, less is more, but a well-placed, simple, acknowledgment of the generosity of people who contributed to your project will make it an unforgettable experience for them.

Adding Photographs to Presentations

If there are members of the group who assisted you along the way, consider adding a photograph of work you did together, with their permission, to engage the audience. If there isn't anyone directly involved, consider including an opening image of people who are affected by the change or participated in the change. When I am taking a photograph I plan to use for publication or dissemination and the subjects are adults, I will announce my intention and ask anyone who does not want to be in the photo to move out of the frame. Then I ask the people in the photo to fill out a consent-for-photography form (can be done online or hard copy) listing their email address so I can send them a copy of the photo. There has never been any objection to any photograph I have taken and shown to other groups. If you are offering an incentive to be in the photograph, I often use a red clown nose as an incentive, give the gift to everyone, even those who are not going to be in the photograph.

If something happens and the photograph you take can't be used or no one agrees to have his or her photograph taken (this has happened on international trips), stage a photograph that demonstrates what you are describing. One photograph is worth a thousand words. And no one wants to hear a thousand words when they can see a photograph.

When children are the focus of the project, include a consent-for-photography form in the instructions or paperwork related to the project. Even with a signed consent, I ask the parent for an email address and the name of the child so they can receive a copy of the photo; I also tell them where the photograph is being submitted. You never know whether the photograph will actually be used, so be sure to say "submitted" if you are disseminating your work to a public media outlet. I've done dozens of children's events and never had a parent object to his or her child's photo being taken when the children are shown in their best light.

Translating Complex Information

Take the long view of your presentation when planning what to include and how to describe specialized information. Following the guidelines in Chapters 20 and 22 for keeping slides and videos uncluttered, remember that certain items should not appear in your presentation. They are:

- Acronyms used without a full spelling of the term
- Graphics with multiple levels of complexity
- Graphics with multiple colors that are essential to understand the meaning of the content
- Information without an example of its significance or application in life
- Games that track points
- Gifts thrown into the audience; this greatly detracts from the substance of your presentation, the content becomes less memorable than the thrown gift

Certain items should always be included:

- Tell a story about the topic. Refer to Chapter 5 on storytelling. The entire presentation should have a beginning, a middle, and an end. The beginning can offer the story of how you came to explore the topic; end with how your life has changed as a result.
- Social media hashtags, even if you are not using one, others may want to talk about it
- Your name and affiliation
- An email or social media account not tied to your job or university as it may be years before someone connects with you and, if you have graduated or changed jobs, the person will not be able to find you
- A statement about conflicts of interest, whether or not any exist
- A statement indicating whether you received any funding for the project
- A selected reference list with only the most important references; you can use the final slide of the presentation for the references
- Refer to everyone by using his or her vocational title (e.g., "doctor") no matter how familiar you are with the people you are referencing

Setting Up the Presentation

Let the audience know whether you will ask for an evaluation and how you will handle questions. Let them know the structure of what will happen and what will be expected of them, then follow that description. If you have a tendency to go off topic, script your presentation. No matter what, stick to your time slot. Never go over the time allotted.

Involving the Audience

There are many ways in which you can involve the audience. Structure their participation based on the time you have available; a general guide is that for every 15 minutes there are two very brief interactions. Here are some suggestions for involving large crowds in 15-minute presentations.

You can do an assessment of what the audience already knows by using a polling technology that can be used with smart phones, such as PollEverywhere.com or use a Google survey. You can also give the audience index cards with two different colors that have a meaning for questions you will be asking that will be used to indicate their answers.

A second activity can reinforce your content. A simple option is to ask members to turn to the person sitting to their right or left and describe one action they will use as a result of your presentation.

Acknowledgments

Save all of the acknowledgments of people who helped you until the end of your presentation. To efficiently recognize people, ask those who are present to stand; others you can indicate through photographs in your presentation. Each method takes just a few seconds and does not take time away from the content.

☐ Archiving Your Presentation

The best way to make your presentation available is to upload it to your blog or website. If you do not have one, use SlideShare as a repository of all your presentations. Then you can direct the audience to the virtual location of the presentation. You may need to remove personally identifying information, such as your phone number or email address, which will not be available in the future if people want to contact you. It is best to use your personal email, Twitter, or other social media. Assume people will want to contact you. Plan ahead with what goes on the Internet.

☐ Conclusions

Presentations can be intimidating and exhilarating. When you are presenting about a topic that you feel very close to, like your capstone project, you may feel vulnerable because you are close to the topic. Most people are going to be very enthusiastic and supportive. For the few people who may take issue with some part of your presentation, remember that if they don't know you personally, there is no reason to take their comments personally. Preparation, practice, patience, and professionalism are the universal ingredients of a successfully disseminated project.

EXHIBIT 26.1 Transcript of a 10-Minute Presentation on My Nursing Model the Silver Hour

On a particularly difficult weekend when I was working on a per diem basis for a hospice, there were a lot of deaths. For me, "a lot" means three or more. Each death went as well as can be expected for a holiday weekend that included per diem staff (me) and on-call physicians not familiar with the patients I was calling about.

Each death went according to the very best of my ability, which was considerable given years of experience in hospice and education. But things were still missing. Each family expressed frustration that certain events did not occur. Being a per diem nurse, I did not know the nicknames of patients, for example. I didn't know the names of beloved pets. I sat in the wrong chair a couple of times. Nothing that was earth shaking, but actions that told the families I was not an insider. I did not know the patients' personal stories. And because it was a holiday weekend and staffing was low, I was busy, I did not have time to listen to the family stories that meant so much to them.

As I left each home and drove to the next, I grew increasingly frustrated. I knew I was not meeting the expectations of the families, yet I knew I was doing my best. But things were not right. Then it hit me, the best idea of my life.

I thought about the effectiveness of the concept of the "golden hour." The golden hour was first described in 2011 and refers to standardizing the care given to people who have suffered a life-threatening event. The golden hour includes actions such as rapid transfer to a trauma center, specialized care, and implementation of disease-specific protocols.

I thought to myself, "we need a golden hour at the time of death." Because the term *golden hour* was already taken, the silver hour seemed appropriate.

As a result, I have developed a flexible model of end-of-life care called the *Silver Hour*. It is the metaphorical last hour of life divided into three time periods: premortem, mortem, and postmortem. Each period has a set of evidence-based actions for the clinical staff to take to ensure the patient and family's needs are placed at the center of the plan of care.

In the premortem phase, the family and patient are told that death is near, the room is marked as a room where someone is dying, and the environment of care is kept as quiet as possible.

The mortem phase involves pronouncing the patient as dead. The person's face is never covered up, the patient is cleaned for the family to view, and the patient is referred to by name.

The postmortem phase is the time immediately after the patient is pronounced dead and removed from the facility. The patient is still considered a patient and staffing reflects the resources needed to provide respectful care to the patient and family; the family is walked to the car and discharge or after-death instructions are given to the family.

The model is used all over the world in nursing education and in any facility, in whole or in pieces. Complete information is available on my website: SilverHour.info.

CHAPTER 27

Your Nursing Career and Continually Building on the First Step

☐ Chapter Checklist

☑	Know your state's requirements for ongoing education
☑	Specialty certification
☑	Journal clubs
☑	Mentoring

Advancing your career through ongoing continuing education (CE) is an integral part of the life of an advanced practice nurse and is required for the maintenance of licenses and certifications as well as career advancement. Make a specific plan for yourself. Don't rely on advancements that are offered to you. Seek out what you want and make it happen (Table 27.1).

☐ Required Continuing Education

CE is not only a good idea for purposes of maintaining up-to-date professional knowledge, but is also a required part of maintaining state practicing license in some states and for some certifications. Every state and territory has a nurse practice act (NPA), which is maintained by the state board of nursing. It is essential for nurses at all levels to be familiar with their state's NPA (which can vary by

TABLE 27.1 Resources for Lifelong Learning and Development

Benner's Novice to Expert Self-Assessment Tool	http://napnapcareerguide.com
American Nurses Association list of nursing organizations	http://nurse.org/orgs.shtml
American Nurses Credentialing Center	http://nursecredentialing.org

state) as it outlines the scope of practice and various requirements, including CE requirements. CEs that are accredited to meet these minimum requirements come in the form of webinars, conferences, and online courses such as those offered by the American Nurses Association (ANA) and by the American Association of Nurse Practitioners (AANP).

☐ Professional Organizations

Being involved with professional organizations can address multiple career topics such as providing a source of CE, networking, mentoring, field-related news, and access to journals. Involvement in associations can result in leadership opportunities as well as involvement in advancement within the profession that is not associated with your employer.

☐ Specialty Certification

One way of advancing nursing careers and lifelong learning habits is to pursue a specialty certification. The American Nurses Credentialing Center (ANCC) offers advanced practice registered nurses (APRNs) advanced certifications in several specialties, including pediatrics, psychiatric/mental health, home health, and more. The ANCC claims that certification increases salaries as well as chances of landing jobs. Renewal of ANCC certifications involves maintaining CE contact hours.

☐ Journal Clubs

In addition to state- and national-level organizations, there are more local means through which APRNs can network with health care professionals that also involve continued learning. Journal clubs, for example, facilitate professionals coming together to work on projects of shared interest by studying the literature. Journal clubs might review a specific research study and discuss implications of the study for clinical practice. Journal clubs encourage continual learning in a professional group setting. They are typically set up as local, physical groups; however, recently journal clubs have appeared on Twitter as well.

☐ Mentoring

A study from the *Journal of Organizational Behavior* states that "mentored individuals reported having more satisfaction, career mobility/opportunity, recognition and a higher promotion rate than non-mentored individuals." APRNs seeking a mentor relationship may use a matching program, such as the one offered by the American Organization of Nurse Executives (AONE) called *Leader2Leader* (www.aone.org/resources/community.shtml). However, a more informal approach can also be taken. A collection of suggestions for advancing your career is at www.nursingjobs.com/five-tips-for-advancing-your-nursing -career. Among the suggestions are to build and use a network and always act professionally.

☐ Self-Assessment

The National Association of Pediatric Nurse Practitioners recommends the use of the Benner novice-to-expert model for the self-assessment of health care professionals' skill levels (Benner, 1982). This model describes five stages from novice to expert: novice, advanced beginner, competent, proficient, expert. APRNs may use this Benner's tool (see Table 27.1) to determine which category they fall in based on their clinical abilities and emotions.

☐ Conclusions

APRNs planning for lifelong learning should familiarize themselves with the minimum CE requirements for maintaining state licenses. They should seriously consider the advantages of joining national and state professional organizations as well as pursuing specialized certification. Participation in local or online learning groups, such as a journal club, can help to maintain up-to-date knowledge, and a mentor relationship can provide career perspective and advice. The use of a self-assessment tool, such as the Benner model, can also advise APRNs of their educational needs as they advance from novice to expert.

REFERENCE

Benner, P. (1982). From novice to expert. *American Journal of Nursing, 82*(3), 402–407.

CHAPTER 28

Career Planning: Using the Work to Further Your Career

☐ Chapter Checklist

☑	Plan how to apply your new skills in your clinical agency.
☑	Keep your résumé current.
☑	Meet with agency leadership to inform them of your new skills.
☑	Create a habit of updating your résumé regularly.

You have taken a short walk across a stage to graduate with your DNP degree while simultaneously blowing apart the walls, floor, and ceiling of your previous boundaries. Once you have recovered from the work of completing your degree and put all the textbooks and project tools away, its time to begin again with a reassessment of how you will build the career you want and deserve.

☐ Applying Your Degree in the Clinical Setting

Along with a doctoral degree (doesn't that sound great?), you now have a chance to apply a wide range of skills across your professional and personal lives. These skills are unique to you and your educational journey. As you finish your degree, it is important to carefully document the significant talents, skills, and experiences you have developed in a résumé. Although résumés are generally one or two pages long, you can develop a longer version in which you have more detail. The length depends on whether you are searching for a job (for which the shorter one would be appropriate) or want to educate leaders about new activities you have been engaged in within your job role (which would call for the longer version). Your manager may not have any detailed idea of the depth and scope of what you know, so you will want to make an appointment and share your new skills and insights with your superiors, even if you are not applying for a new job. Publicize yourself and your readiness to take on new challenges. Be specific about what you are looking for in your next challenge.

Current Résumé

During the process of completing your capstone project, be sure to keep careful records of what you did and who assisted you. Be especially careful about what was done while you were being paid by your employer and what you did as a student. Wearing a student name tag is very helpful when distinguishing between your roles. Many people will be involved in your capstone project. It is critical that your description of what you did is clear and correct. Everyone who contributed in meaningful ways should be given credit for what his or her contribution. Periodically check in with others in your group to make sure any contracts or group guidelines you made were followed. If not, were they amended? Make sure you include a record of what you have done and how it has contributed to the people around you and the organization you work for. A portfolio you turned in for your university is not appropriate for use with your employer. Your university has specific accreditation standards that are different than those for a clinical agency. Knowing your audience is the first rule of making a presentation. Show work samples that are relevant to your employer. The OWL Purdue Writing lab provides an online guide for writing a resume (https://owl.english.purdue.edu/owl/resource/564/1).

Routinely Update Résumé

Maintaining an accurate work history of committees, projects, and education will assist you in preparing for performance evaluations. This record-keeping is often overlooked by many nurses who are uncomfortable promoting themselves and feel it takes too much time. However, if you do not showcase your newly acquired talents and accomplishments, no one will. Use all the tools and strategies you learned in this text to provide others with inspiration to follow in your footsteps as a lifelong learner and to step outside their comfort zone as you have.

You can keep an electronic calendar and a file folder that contains announcements of meetings and other relevant activities. Then periodically review this and use it to update your résumé. Regularly reviewing your accomplishments has to become a habit. This habit will help you be ready for promotions, new challenges, and other experiences.

Curriculum Vitae (CV)

A CV favors educational and scholarly information as it is related more to academic jobs than clinical. It is a detailed document and may have a different layout and headings. Typical headings on a CV are: educational or mentoring work you do with students and presentation and publications (including your project). A great reference for composing a CV is at the OWL Purdue writing lab (https://owl.english.purdue.edu/owl/resource/641/1).

☐ Conclusions

Letting people know what you've learned and how your view of yourself as a clinician has changed is important. Once the dust settles after you finish your degree, make an appointment to speak with someone in a leadership position in your organization, someone who is likely to be in a position to be a mentor who can assist you to move to the next level. Have a meeting even if you are content with your current role; there are always opportunities to work on projects and effect change in different ways. Let others know you are ready. Be able to show them you are ready with a current résumé that is clear, concise, and focused on what the reader is looking for. You may need to create several versions. The point is to showcase yourself and your amazing accomplishments!

Case Study: Cindy Fike, DNP

☐ Personal Journey

As a graduate of the charter class of the first DNPs to successfully complete the program in Southern California, myself and all the graduates were mentored and taught by professors with PhDs. The graduating defense was called the *clinical dissertation*, with the expectation that one or more of the university faculty or review boards would be in attendance at the presentation. Upon successful defense of the "clinical dissertation" the DNP was encouraged by the professors to publish their work. The majority of DNPs did not publish their work as many of the graduates were advanced practice nurses and/or hospital leaders with goals of applying research into practice. A handful of graduates were from academia; one of the graduates became a chair of a local college, another taught at a university in Canada, whereas the other two were professors at local universities.

Although DNP students/graduates attempt to enter the academic arena, they are faced with questions regarding their publications. The DNP student/graduate usually does not contemplate publishing unless necessitated by an occupation requirement.

Another DNP candidate was successful in defending his "clinical dissertation" and awarded his DNP. He did not think of publishing his work on surgical outcomes and core measures because he was working as an informatics specialist for a large not-for-profit organization. He works in a nursing registry in the med–surg unit on the weekends and 2 years later decided to apply for a tenured-track position at the university. He was not hired because of his lack of publications. The best advice for any DNP is to publish her or his work; many want to know how to get their first work published. With changes to careers and goals for the DNP, they are now looking for scholarly mentoring and asking many of questions regarding research and publishing.

Another nurse practitioner (NP) DNP did not publish after graduation and, although working as an NP for 10 years in the emergency department, has decided to take a tenured-track position at the university; this DNP is now asking the same questions regarding research and publishing.

Both DNPs had their graduation work in a bound book and approved as publishable, as required by the DNP program. Yet they had their books on a shelf, never thinking they would change to careers in which publication is required.

Many issues and concerns present challenges to current DNPs in first-time academic positions including, but not limited to, how to edit, what journals to select, what is a primary investigator, learning better writing skills, finding the time to write, setting goals, and so forth. Also, many new DNPs in a new tenured-track position may find themselves in a role in which they don't know what they don't know, therefore making it difficult to ask the right questions. The new tenured-track academic must find mentoring within and outside of the department and college. Mentoring from past professors can be a great resource; the DNP must be assertive in finding a mentor.

In reviewing the expectations of "The DNP Charter Class Clinical Dissertation Guidelines," the 16 components, which appeared to be relative to the success of the students who chose the academia path, included:

1. Clinical dissertation chair
2. Clinical dissertation committee approval
3. Termination of clinical dissertation chair relationship
4. Termination of clinical dissertation committee members
5. Clinical dissertation proposal approval
6. Institutional Review and Approval
7. Proposal approval form
8. Conducting the project
9. Approval of the clinical dissertation
10. Clinical dissertation oral defense
11. Order of the defense
12. Determination of success or failure of defense
13. Repeating the oral defense
14. Submission of final clinical dissertation
15. Binding of clinical dissertation
16. Components of the clinical dissertation

Much work and effort was developed and accomplished by these DNP graduates; they were given the recommendations to find a profession mentor and guide, including the recommendation to go beyond the final project as an evidence-based practice application-oriented final DNP project and try to publish their work, especially as research will become a focus in the academia arena for those seeking employment as faculty members.

☐ Personal Take

I should probably change this title to "frustration" as this is what I have experienced and what I hear from the majority of DNP colleagues who are now faced with having to publish as a requirement of their newly acquired position in academia.

This year I served as part of the search committee at the university and the question posed by the committee when reviewing applicants was "has the applicant been published?" Of course, the applicant would not have published anything unless he or she did so as part of previous employment that required publication for tenured-track purposes. Most DNPs who presented their research during the interview offered a project, which seems to lack the luster and backbone of a PhD research presentation when seeking employment in academia.

As a newly hired tenured-track assistant professor myself, I was frustrated with what appear to be daily obstacles in finding an appropriate path to publication.

The following are some of the trials and tribulations encountered (mind you, I had to research many of these items to clarify their meaning):

- Different input given by professors as to what will work/what won't work
- Don't publish in an open access journal/do publish in an open access journal
- Only publish with a journal that has an impact factor/it doesn't matter if the journal has an impact factor (what's an impact factor?)
- An internal grant is a must/An external grant is a must (how to write a grant for the first time?)
- Biosketch?
- Letter of intent?
- Pedagogy, how best to apply, teach, publish
- Worked on a first article and was rejected by a journal
- Worked on a second article and was rejected by a journal
- Never heard back from one journal
- I didn't know what I didn't know
- The amount of time it takes to publish
- Publish alone or with others?
- Stay focused on my dissertation area
- Don't waste time writing a book
- Don't overextend yourself/Keep your plate full
- Institutional review board committee review is needed by the university
- Grant submission made from a central person through the university
- Finding time to research, write, etc.
- Staying on track and organized

Conflicting advice on how to get published has probably been the most difficult. Remember, although I had limited exposure to one potential publishable article (my dissertation), the rest of my experience is from workshops, colleagues, advice received, and so on The first time I submitted my revised article generated from my dissertation for publication and was rejected, the feeling was of plain disappointment. This is probably because I didn't understand the process and that all professors are rejected at some time. A retired professor advised me to send my dissertation to an online library of research and information. The advice from this retired professor was that the dissertation was considered to be my first publication. Although, among the conflicting advice, yet another professor told me this was not the case. I submitted another article to an online journal, which did not have an impact factor but was accepted for publication. This international journal reaches all nurses, which to me is a success. Another professor who has taken me under her wing also guided me along the path and recently an article we wrote jointly was published.

What works and what I have learned:

- My writing is my most important strength.
- I need to surround myself with mentors, tenured professors, and those committed to publishing.
- I must attend as many workshops and conferences as possible and ask questions, although the questions may not come for a while.
- It is essential to stay focused. It is so easy to be absorbed by learning how to be a professor.
- Skills learned from past employment can be very valuable when working toward publication.

I will soon complete my second year of teaching. I am slowly progressing on a new path from "I don't know what I don't know" to "I know what I don't know" and I won't stop or give up.

SHARED Model Template

Model	Inputs	Outputs
Select	Topic Broad area Visuals	Finding sources of artwork in the public domain to use (some offer photos for a few, too): Ancestry Images: ancestryimages.com Norway's National Museum: samling.nasjonalmuseet.no/en Stock Up: sitebuilderreport.com/stock-up (search multiple sites in one place) crowthestone.com designerspics.com dreamstime.com everystockphoto.com finda.photo freeimages.com freephotosbank.com goodfreephotos.com imcreator.com/free morguefile.com National Gallery of Art: images.nga.gov/ennos.tw nsnd.co photoeverywhere.co.uk pickupimage.com picjumbo.com pixabay.com public-domain-photos.com skitterphoto.com splashbase.co startupstockphotos.com unsplash.com wikiart.org

(continued)

Model	Inputs	Outputs
		Look in all museums and archives; generally, their collection of art is digitized and freely available for educational purposes Welcome Trust: wellcome.ac.uk The Getty: www.getty.edu Munch Museum: emunch.no National Aeronautics and Space Administration archive (also on Flickr): archive.org/details/nasa Project Apollo Archive: flickr.com/photos/projectapolloarchive National Gallery of Art: nga.gov/content/ngaweb.html Pablo: buffer.com/pablo Smithsonian: www.flickr.com/photos/smithsonian **Screenshot makers** awesomescreenshot.com snagit.com PrtScr button on keyboard Skitch **Handouts, posters, and digital graphics can easily be created with a great tool:** Be Funky: befunky.com canva.com iPhoto (Mac) Paint (Windows) Photovisi: photovisi.com picmonkey.com pixlr.com Timeline Slicer: timelineslicer.com **Logo** logogarden.com logotypemaker.com **Social media** easycovermaker.com pagemodo.com/welcome/cover-photos profilepicturemaker.com **Infographics** canva.com infoactive.co Infogram: infogr.am piktochart.com venngage.com visual.ly

Model	Inputs	Outputs
		Pictures with quotes pinwords.com Quozio: quozio.com Recite: recitethis.com/ **Word clouds** tagzedo.com wordclouds.com worditout.com wordle.com **Animated gif maker** ezgif.com/maker gifcreator.me gifmaker.me phhhoto.com **Memes** memegenerator.net/create/generator imgflip.com/memegenerator **Additional sources of information** Free Technology For Teachers: freetech4teachers.com Doug Off the Record: dougpete.wordpress.com Creative Commons Licensing: http://creativecommons.org If you have an image and are not sure whether you are legally entitled to use it, search the image in Google and you will find the usage rights. Be sure to rename images with your name and other keyword. ALWAYS give attribution for work you use created by others, even if not required. Even though these images are "free," it takes money to keep these sites up and available to us. Always show your gratitude by making a donation to your favorite sites, "like" them, leave positive feedback, comment and share in your social media accounts.

(continued)

Model	Inputs	Outputs
Habits	**Collect evidence** Online databases Guidelines, practice standards Social media Arts: music, literature, painting Multimedia	
Assess	**Timeliness** Program deadlines Project schedule **Budget communication** Face-to-face Video conferencing Telephone Texting	
Assess	Content knowledge Develop skills for acquiring existing knowl-edge—search-ing library and Internet Technical knowledge	
Record	Soft notes—temporary, handwritten, local files, online User names and passwords Budget Progress to-ward program	Evernote Google Calendar Google Drive Wikis Paper and pencil

Model	Inputs	Outputs
Enthusiasm	Keep the project realistic. Ensure that you have the resources to complete the project or a plan to get the resources. Take care of yourself. Take a break when you need to. Be honest with yourself and others throughout the process.	Keep a journal. Socialize with colleagues and team members who are supporting your efforts. Say "thank you." Share the credit when appropriate.
Disseminate	Disseminating means considering all the possibilities of giving others access to your project details. Strategies can include publications, videos, microblogs, or artistic products.	

Index

Note: Page numbers followed by f and t denotes figures and tables respectively.

CPSIA information can be obtained
at www.ICGtesting.com
Printed in the USA
BVHW041800071220
595105BV00008B/133